THE
MONDAY
TO FRIDAY
DIET

THE
MONDAY
TO FRIDAY
DIET

LOSE WEIGHT
& ENJOY YOUR WEEKEND

SUSIE BURRELL

SYD   NDON

A Bantam book
Published by Random House Australia Pty Ltd
Level 3, 100 Pacific Highway, North Sydney NSW 2060
www.randomhouse.com.au

First published by Bantam in 2013

Addresses for companies within the Random House Group can be found at
ıwww.randomhouse.com.au/offices

National Library of Australia
Cataloguing-in-Publication entry (pbk.)

Burrell, Susie.
The Monday to Friday diet / Susie Burrell.

ISBN 978 1 74275 521 2 (pbk.)

Body weight – Regulation.
Reducing diets.
Weight loss.

613.25

Cover illustration courtesy iStockphoto/Keith Bishop
Author photo by Brendan Ralph
Cover design by Cathie Glassby
Internal design and typesetting by Midland Typesetters, Australia
Printed in Australia by Griffin Press, an accredited ISO AS/NZS 14001:2004
Environmental Management System printer

*For anyone who has battled their way through a bleak
12-hour work day, may this book help you to regain
control over your health, your body and your life.*

*Written in loving memory of our boy Henry, who brought
us so much joy — you are always in our thoughts.*

CONTENTS

Introduction: The Monday to Friday Diet

Over the past 13 years, through my work as a specialist weight-loss dietitian, I have seen hundreds of smart, successful, focused clients who, despite their numerous achievements, struggle to get their weight under control amid the chaos in which they live. Working hours are long, stress is high and, although they theoretically 'know' what they 'should' be doing to keep their weight under control, their busyness makes it nearly impossible.

The Monday to Friday Diet was written to share with you the tricks and tips I use in practice with my own clients to help them structure their working week in a way that is conducive to weight control. The specific diet plans for each day of the week, which alter according to caloric intake, ease of preparation and food density, support weight control no matter what the demands of the day may be. *The Monday to Friday Diet* will help you look at each weekday with specific diet and exercise goals in mind. It allows you to indulge a little more on weekends and have a 'reset' day to regain control after the typical weekend festivities, and it links quick-and-easy, calorie-controlled recipes to the busier days of the week. Such a structure is not only helpful when it comes to losing weight, but it will help you get organised and take control of your food intake – no matter how busy you are.

As the title suggests, *The Monday to Friday Diet* is a 'diet' but, rather than a regime that you need to follow strictly to get results, the program is designed to give you a structure within which to base your food intake on any specific day of the week, which in turn will help to control your caloric intake throughout the course of a week and help prevent the weight-loss/weight-gain cycle. The recipes that accompany each day vary in both caloric and carbohydrate content, which means that they are each suited to their specific days. There is also a range of tricks, tips and ideas throughout the entire plan that are likely to benefit you and your weight-loss goals on any given day of the week.

It is my goal to help my clients develop their *own* skills to help manage their *own* working weeks, and it is my hope that *The Monday to Friday Diet* offers you the very same support. Once we a have a clear structure on any given day of the week, where we know what we need to do as a minimum to stay on track, we are also able to manage our food intake and exercise habits to support our health and fitness goals. Once we reach this point, we can ultimately take control of our weight, for good.

This week is going to be different to all the others; this is going to be the week I get my food, my diet and my life on track, once and for all.

Why weekdays?

How many times in your life have you started your week with the best diet intentions? Of 'being good' this week and beginning your low-carb regime and getting to the gym every day – of this week being different from the hundreds or thousands of others that you have already lived. This is the week you will finally make major inroads into becoming the weight, shape and size you have always wanted to be.

Unfortunately for many of us, by Wednesday, or even lunchtime Monday, these thoughts and declarations are old news. Work and life have taken over again and we are back to where we started on Monday – feeling fat, unfit and overwhelmed.

We tend to feel this way because many of us have become slaves to our work and the Monday-to-Friday grind. Long working days with hours spent commuting and a constantly over-scheduled, frantic lifestyle mean that we eat too much, too often. Plus we eat high-fat, high-sugar foods to reward ourselves for being at work, and we move our bodies far, far less than they need to be moved.

While we may start working in our 20s, when we are relatively slim and in control of our weight, a 5–10kg weight gain gradually accumulates throughout our 30s, which can translate into an extra 20kg or even 30kg gain over the 20 or more years we spend in the workforce. And, in many cases, this has happened without us even noticing. Work drinks, celebratory cakes, the office biscuit tin, processed foods eaten in front of the computer and unforgiving work hours leave us with little time to cook, exercise or achieve the elusive work–life balance.

Unfortunately for us, our metabolism is not so forgiving, and once any extra weight is there it stays there – whether 5kg or 30kg, it is very hard to lose. And while good intentions on a Monday morning are fabulous, they are simply not enough to save us from our work–weight-gain cycle.

The fact that our careers are so important to us and we spend so much time working means that we need to take into account the challenges of the week when we plan for successful weight loss. Incorporating our work and life commitments into any diet and exercise regime is crucial in not only helping us develop a sustainable lifestyle framework but also in ensuring that our Monday morning intentions ultimately become second nature throughout our working life. These habits will allow us to strike a balance between having a good time on the weekend and compensating through the week; to be prepared for the ups and downs of the working week and adjust our food intake accordingly; and to help us remain in control of our weight rather than being a victim of it.

And, hence, the reason why *The Monday to Friday Diet* has been written: to serve as a guide to teach you how to structure your week so that your food and lifestyle choices come together to support weight loss. To learn that much of the effort we need to put in to control our weight is actually completed on Sunday. To know how to structure your Mondays in a way that will ensure your diet and exercise are on track until midweek; and how to compensate for a big weekend or a work dinner out. To have the knowledge and skill set to be able to create the space in your week to recharge and reset your food and exercise so that you again feel in control and on track of your food, your body and your life. To know exactly what to eat and when throughout the week so you can still enjoy your food but keep your calories under control. And perhaps most importantly, to know what to eat so you can compensate when you have overdone things.

For all of us, weight loss comes down to individual decisions on a daily basis about what we will eat and when and how we will move. Once we have these decisions linked to the structure of our working weeks, our food, exercise and energy improve, which can help life become a whole lot easier.

Why weekdays are so tough

❀ *People lose weight when they are removed from the demands of day-to-day life – as soon as life returns to normal, things become a little more complicated.*

Modern life is tough; not only do we have intense demands on our time and resources but when it comes to our health and fitness, we constantly find ourselves battling silent but powerful enemies. These enemies can be the environment, the people we spend our time with including friends and family, and work itself. But until we identify our diet and exercise saboteurs and manage them, taking control of our food, our bodies and our lives will continually prove challenging. The good news is that the simple act of identifying our own potential diet and exercise enemies and developing clear management plans for them will ultimately keep us on track with our personal health and wellbeing goals.

Work

Most of us have to work, some of us may even really enjoy it, but the truth is that the confinements of the working day, whether we work 9 to 5 Monday to Friday, shiftwork or casually at a local store or restaurant, rarely tend to be of help when it comes to weight control. Whether it is the time we spend getting there, the stress of the work itself, the people we work with or the long hours, the working day can see us eat far more than we need, be exposed to foods that we never usually would and have us miss our training session or gym class simply because we run out of time.

Now, of course, when it comes to going to work and earning a living, no one is saying that we cannot work and keep our weight under control at the same time, but it is important that we remain aware of the challenges that work imposes on our lifestyle choices so we are able to develop strategies for coping with these limitations on a daily basis. In an ideal world, we would all have flexible working hours, gyms at work, healthy foods and snacks on hand, and workplaces that supported health, fitness and wellbeing 100%. Indeed, some workplaces do offer this, but until this scenario is the norm, we all have to work hard to make the best of whatever work situation we find ourselves in. The harsh reality is that if we don't, our health, wellbeing and relationships are ultimately what will suffer.

Colleagues

The people we work with may be well-meaning people who we love spending time with, or they may be people we can easily work with but we would never spend time with on the weekends, or they may be people we simply cannot stand. Chances are, they are a mix of these three groups of people and just as we did at school, we will like and prefer the company of some workmates over others. Now, whether we like them or not is largely irrelevant here; all we need to be aware of are the small but significant ways in which they can influence our food habits on a daily basis.

Research indicates that in general we become like the people we spend our time with, so if your colleagues regularly indulge in high-fat fast food at work, snack often, drink much coffee, eat at their desks and rarely leave the office during the working day, statistics would suggest that you will adopt at least some of these habits long term. On the other hand, if everyone at your workplace stops for lunch, people eat only at mealtimes, celebrate special occasions with food once a month instead of once a week and promote physical activity, chances are that you are going to be a whole lot healthier.

Once you have identified that you are committed to weight control, managing the potential influence your colleagues' food habits have on you is crucial. Just as we need to manage our relationships to maintain boundaries and self-respect, so too do we need to do this with our colleagues, no matter how well-meaning they may seem. At times this will mean saying no to extra cakes and biscuits, being the only person who does not participate in pizza day, or going for a lunchtime run when everyone else is working through their lunch-break. But, ultimately, it will also mean that you are healthier and happier as a result.

Friends

Managing your own behaviour in the company of others is one thing, but being able to do it in the company of those closest to you is a whole other story. While our friends are often the people we turn to for support and guidance on a daily basis, they can also have a huge influence over the way we behave, particularly in terms of what we eat and how much we move. How many times can you remember vowing not to drink alcohol, or have dessert, only to be convinced to indulge a little by well-meaning friends who simply feel more comfortable doing these things themselves if you are doing it with them?

The other issue that arises with weekdays is that we not only deal with the influence of colleagues but also the influence of friends, who we may meet for lunch, plan to go to the gym with, shop with at lunchtime or meet after work for a drink. These social influences add up, and before we know it our diet and training plans have been derailed several times in a single day.

The first step towards making sure that your friendship influences are positive rather than a hindrance in your quest for weight control is to become aware of the ways in which these interactions can be both positive and negative. Once we are aware of the ways in which daily decisions start to impact the long-term goals we have for ourselves, it becomes easier to make the necessary adjustments and changes and move forward. In the case of friends, this may mean altering the context in which you see them, stating your goals clearly, or even communicating the ways in which the interaction is hampering your attempts at weight control so your friends can make the choice to support you or not.

The environment

People come and go in our workday lives on a daily basis but the environment in which we find ourselves can play a massive role in influencing our energy levels, motivation and ability to eat well and look after our bodies. In more cases than not, the workplace environment is less than ideal and may require some serious changes or mental reframing to ensure it is conducive to weight control.

The toxic work environment

❀ *Is your office an inspiring workplace or a cave in which bad habits breed?*

While it is the norm for a great number of people, the truth is that sitting at a desk, with no natural air or sunlight, and minimal movement for at least 8 hours each day, is not good for us. In fact, for many of us, it is the very reason why we are constantly feeling tired, run-down and overwhelmed. As you can imagine, when you are not feeling 100% it can be exceptionally challenging to get through the day, let alone to fully focus and commit to a healthy lifestyle.

The toxicity of a work environment is generated via numerous pathways. Research has shown that working in close proximity to others means that we become vulnerable to picking up their habits simply because human beings will naturally 'become like the people they spend their time with'. Offices are notorious for giving easy access to high-calorie, energy-dense foods, whether via the fundraising chocolate box or office biscuit jar. Then we have the sad fact that there are people who actually do not like being at work very much and self-reward with food just to get through the day. And this is only a surface look at factors that contribute to make the office environment a diet and wellbeing nightmare – there are a few more common issues.

The office kitchen

You may be one of the lucky few whose office has access to pristine kitchen facilities but in general, the office kitchen is not up to the hygiene standards that you try to maintain at home. Not only does the unhygienic environment make it far more appealing to purchase your food rather than prepare it at work, it also means that you are less likely to leave your desk to eat and enjoy your food in the work kitchen at mealtimes.

Or, sometimes the kitchen is simply a major risk to your healthy lifestyle, because it is where the biscuits, celebratory cakes and fundraising chocolates are at hand's reach. Or it is the scene of an occasional 3pm raid in the past, times when you have literally done whatever you have needed to do in order to get your hands on something sweet.

Unless you are one of the lucky few who have a company that fully caters for the staff, or whose cleaners are particularly good, in most cases the office kitchen is a space to be very wary of.

Staff celebrations

How often is there a birthday, an engagement, a new baby, or someone leaving to celebrate during the working week? In some workplaces cakes and treats occur so often that you are more likely to eat cake on any given day than not. This is all well and good, but if we then go home and celebrate various family and other social events, we can be eating cake and other sweet treats multiple times every week. And heaven forbid if you say no to a piece of cake, because then it is likely that a colleague will make it their priority to ensure that you eat it, no matter what.

There is nothing wrong with enjoying treats occasionally, but in many cases 'occasionally' becomes almost every day, and that is at least an extra 200–300 calories a week that we really do not need.

The biscuit jar

At face value, the willingness of our employers to provide us with various refreshments to help us get through the working day is a kind gesture, but unfortunately the most common options of biscuits and confectionery are far from ideal. Not only do such foods offer us little nutritionally, they are also foods that are exceptionally easy to overeat and that we are easily tempted by when we go to the kitchen to make a cup of tea or coffee. Research has shown that we are likely to eat double the number of sweet treats when we can see them. So, for this reason, keeping the biscuit or lolly jar well hidden when we are at work is crucial if we are to stay well away from these tasty workday treats, which can become nasty food habits if we are not careful.

Fundraising

We have all been there – purchasing the entire box of fundraising chocolates and then promptly eating them even though we had promised ourselves that we would doorknock the neighbours and flog them off. Just because they are 'for a good cause' does not make them calorie-free, and fundraising chocolates also tend to be significantly larger than regular chocolate bars and sweet treats. Colleagues who place their box of fundraising chocolates smack bang in the middle of the lunch room table are incredibly smart – they know that desperate work colleagues will do anything for sweet food at 3pm, and even the toughest resolve will find it difficult to resist when they can buy a jumbo chocolate bar for a dollar.

Lunch at your desk

There are two main issues associated with eating at your desk. The first is that if you are eating while you are doing something else you may not be eating mindfully. This means that you are not paying full attention to how much you are eating and are more likely to overeat. Second, sitting at your desk to eat your lunch is likely to mean that you have been sedentary for most of the day, when lunchtime offers the perfect opportunity to go outside and get some sunlight and move your body.

Coffee

If there is one dietary factor that has changed enormously over the past 5 to 10 years, it would be the influence of coffee on our calorie intake. In the 1970s and 80s, coffee was likely to be black with a little milk or sugar, whereas now it tends to be a large or grande packed with milk, sugar and sometimes flavourings. A one-a-day coffee habit is more likely to be replaced with a couple of coffees a day, which often centre on a social outing with other people from the office. Meals are replaced with coffee, the liquid calories are not compensated for and it could be argued that the increasing consumption of milk-based coffee is closely linked to the increasing weight of adults in general. This is particularly so for office workers in which the trip to the coffee shop or cart can be the highlight of the day.

Working long hours

Long gone are the days of 9 to 5, with working hours now more likely to be 8 till 6, and that often counts as an easy day in the office. The increasing length of the working day, without even taking into consideration the commuting times, means that we have less and less time for recreation and exercise. Our days are largely spent sitting, with any spare time shunted towards more work or social activities, which means that many of us barely move all day. The downside of this is that day by day, our metabolic rate slows, which means that on a daily basis we burn fewer and fewer calories and so it is easier and easier to gain weight.

The vending machine

It has happened to all of us: while we start out with the best intentions, on those days in which we are not 100% organised and do not have all our healthy snacks on hand we resort to a sugar hit from the vending machine. When work is intense or we need a quick energy hit out of hours, often the only food option available are high-calorie snack foods bought from local shops and vending machines. Human beings will eat whatever foods are readily available to them, which means that if there is a vending machine in your workplace, chances are you will indulge at times – even if you do not really want to.

Work drinks

For some workplaces, after-work drinks are an occasional event, while for others they are far more frequent, celebrating anything from an account win to simply making it through the week. The issue with combining work with social events is that we find ourselves over-consuming both alcohol and food as part of our weekly work schedule as well as in our social lives. Another issue that presents when socialising and eating with workmates is the feeling of having to 'keep up' with our boss or competitive colleagues, which inevitably means we eat and drink far more than we usually would. As we spend so much time at work, the decisions we make in relation to our food and drink intake have a powerful influence over our health and weight control whether we like it or not.

Workplace 'feeders'

You know exactly who I am talking about: the seemingly well-meaning work colleague who appears to have your best interests at heart but who also seems to be constantly encouraging you to eat more and more. The thing about other people is that, generally speaking, they are thinking about themselves and the way that your eating habits impact on them, as opposed to genuinely considering your health, weight and wellbeing. Dealing with other people, particularly when you are trying to control your calorie intake and stay on track with your diet, may mean that you are going to have to be tough. Keep your own health and fitness goals at the forefront of your mind if you are to prevent getting sidetracked by others' seemingly well-intentioned suggestions that you eat and drink things you would rather not.

How to face reality

In an ideal world, all these factors would be manageable. We would have supportive employers who made it their priority to create a workplace that was conducive to a healthy lifestyle. Office mates too would band together and make a pact to only eat healthy, nutritious food and exercise at lunchtime, and work celebrations would be an occasional social event. Unfortunately, life can be a little more complicated than this, which means if you have identified that you need to make sustainable lifestyle choices to lose weight and keep it off, ultimately these changes are going to have to come from you. Only then will you be able to continue these lifestyle choices when you are at work and dealing with the average working week.

Taking charge of your week

✛ *There will always be distractions, detours,*
roadblocks and excuses, and until we take charge of
them they will always put us off our game.

A crucial aspect of feeling and being in control of our week is accepting that at certain times things will not always go to plan. That is life. But our ability to accept this and move forward without completely sabotaging our weight-loss efforts is paramount to our success. Often we play the victim and say we cannot help it, because this is what we have been taught as children or had habitually programmed into us throughout our adult life. Or we adopt a mental position that if everything is not 'perfect', if we do not stick to our diet 100%, or have one slip-up, we should immediately throw in the towel and wait until the next new and perfect day – which never comes.

Taking charge means moving above and beyond these imposed mental limitations to achieve success. To always doing your best and making the best choices under whatever circumstances are present. To programming your thoughts to always work towards a baseline of positive lifestyle choices and accepting that, at times, things will not always be perfect. Additionally, it means becoming empowered to look for the best choices and feeling confident in doing so, rather than being guided by outside opinions, diets and one-off programs that promise the world but rarely deliver long term.

Once you have shifted towards a mental mindset of 'I can do this', as opposed to constantly feeling challenged, frustrated and out of control, your brain will open up different processing pathways and look for opportunities rather than limitations. The new mindset reiterates the fact that all is not lost when you eat something you should not have eaten, or when you skip a training session, but that all you need to do is get back on track immediately. No more, 'I will start on Monday', or 'it doesn't matter, I have broken my diet now' – do it immediately.

As is the case with all areas of behavioural change, this process does take time, especially if you have followed a range of different diets and weight-loss programs over long periods of time. But to free yourself of the dieting cycle long term, this is the mental space you need to work towards.

Taking charge of your enemies

❀ *Keep your friends close and your enemies closer.*

Your weekday food enemies, whether they are your colleagues, friends or family, are not going anywhere, so they need to be managed. For some of us, this will be easy – if you have a strong mindset and willpower, you will not find it difficult to say no to people and stick to your plan and stay on track with your goals. For others, though, saying no can be extremely difficult. Sometimes we don't really want to say no, but more often than not we simply do not want to upset or offend anyone, so it is easier to accept the slice of cake or the dessert and be done with it.

Unfortunately, in today's environment, where food is readily available and people are looking for ways to minimise movement rather than do more of it, at times we have to be prepared to say no simply to keep on track with our health and lifestyle goals. This may not necessarily be easy, but these skills will be useful to maintain our personal boundaries and goals long term.

ALWAYS KEEP YOUR GOALS AT THE FOREFRONT OF YOUR MIND

There are never-ending opportunities to eat, indulge, over-consume and socialise, and yet we do not have unlimited chances to take control of our weight and the health of our body. Sure, we may be able to lose weight effectively once or twice, but each and every time we gain weight and then try to lose it again, it becomes harder and harder for the body to lose weight. Muscle tone diminishes, as does our metabolic rate and fitness, and we can rarely regain the health, fitness and energy that we once remember having.

For this reason, if we are to keep in control of our weight, for good, we need to constantly keep the health and fitness goals that we have for ourselves at the forefront of our minds. This way we can work towards the right balance of health and fitness for us as individuals and make our daily food and exercise choices based on this.

KNOW YOUR PERSONAL LIMITS

Knowing how to set and keep personal limits and boundaries is imperative in all aspects of life, or we can be left drained, fatigued and frustrated that we have been distracted from our personal goals and pulled into the influence and plans of others. Developing your own personal limits when it comes to your food and drink intake, and the way you allocate time to your training and exercise regimes, is crucial when one of your goals is weight control. Once you know how many times each week you can drink alcohol and not gain weight, or how many gym sessions you need to get to, it becomes easier to map out your week and work towards a balance between your health goals and being social with friends and family.

PRACTISE SAYING NO

Why do we have such problems with saying no? Is it because we do not want to upset or disappoint people? Or is it because we do not know what we want? Or is it simply that it is easier to say yes and deal with the ramifications later? The answer is probably a mix of the three, but when it comes to declining food and drink that we do not really want, or more importantly need, the ability to say no is powerful. And chances are, if you have difficulty saying no to food, you probably also have difficulty saying no to a range of other things that you do not want to do.

The good thing about learning to say no is that it becomes easier. And as is the case with all communication, the more definite you are when you say it, and the more clearly you say it, the more likely it is that your message will get through. There is no need to explain why or offer excuses, such as 'It is just that I am trying to lose weight; I am so sorry but I do not want that cake.' A simple 'no, thank you' is all it will take if you say it the right way.

DIFFERENTIATE BETWEEN 'SPECIAL' AND 'EVERYDAY'

A key technique that may be useful when it comes to weight control is the ability to differentiate between 'special' occasions in which it is completely normal to indulge a little, and day-to-day events in which many of us cannot afford to waste our calories. Once you know if it is a special cake or treat, you can then decide if you will enjoy some, or whether an event is important enough for you to skip the gym to attend it. For each and every one of us, on any particular week, these guidelines will vary, but being clear in your mind of where the event or special occasion fits in the bigger picture of your life will help to guide many of your food decisions on a daily basis.

BE AN INDIVIDUAL IN A COMMUNAL WORLD

Being an individual is perhaps easier said than done because the truth is that human beings like to feel similar to other human beings, which means that when others are eating cake or a friend's homemade pasta or heavy dessert, they want you to as well. In a world that is far from conducive to weight control, making the commitment to eat well and exercise regularly will at times mean that you do need to be different from other people. But ultimately, as an individual, this is a decision you need to make if your weight, health and fitness are to take priority in your world.

Taking charge of your environment

❉ *You can know everything there is to know about nutrition but if your environment is not conducive to eating well, it will be difficult to stay on track.*

IS YOUR HOME A VACUUM FOR A HEALTHY LIFESTYLE?

Healthy people are healthy at home and at work – they develop and keep structures within their world that allow them to maintain a nutritious diet and regular exercise program no matter what demands they have on their time. And this lifestyle begins in the home. Is your kitchen filled with nutritious food? Are your rooms organised and your workout clothes clean and packed away so you can easily find them? Do you keep extra food and treats in your car or handbag? Ensuring that your home is conducive to eating well and exercising is a crucial first step towards committing to health and fitness long term.

THE KITCHEN CLEAN-OUT

If it's in the house, you will eat it. So if you know that your fridge and pantry contain plenty of non-nutritious, high-calorie food choices, it is time to get serious. It does not matter that the treats are 'only for the children' or for 'special occasions' – if you choose to keep tempting foods within easy access at home, and you know that you generally cannot control yourself, you need to throw them away.

BACKUP MEALS

Busy lives mean that there are times when all of us need to rely on quick and easy meal options to get us through a bind. Knowing this, all we need to do to keep on top of things is make it a priority to keep a couple of backup meal options on hand to fill in the gaps on those nights when we are too tired to cook. Frozen vegetables, some leftover healthy meals or soups are all easy to reheat options, and far better nutritionally than a dinner of toast or breakfast cereal.

READY-TO-GO SNACKS

Just as we need to have backup meals on hand to eat well, so too do we need a supply of ready-to-go snacks. In particular, low calories, nutrient dense, filling and portion controlled options are ideal. Fresh vegetables, plain popcorn, wholegrain crackers and thick natural yoghurt all offer the balance of tasting good and being healthy, as opposed to snack bars, biscuits and dried fruit bars and bites.

REGULAR SHOPPING

Whether you do your shopping at lunchtime, online or get a friend to pick up your supplies, if you are not prepared to stock up on healthy dietary staples at least once each week, it is going to be really difficult to eat well. Have a set shopping day and stick to it.

OUT OF SIGHT, OUT OF MIND

Perhaps the most important rule of weight control is that if you do not have food around, and particularly in sight, you are far less likely to eat it. For this reason, keep any biscuits, snacks, fruit and other easy-to-grab foods out of sight when you open the cupboard or pantry at home or even at work, and notice how much more in control of your eating you are when you are not in constant contact with food.

Committing to optimising energy

> ❁ *The mental, physical, emotional and spiritual energy we generate for ourselves is limitless, if we know how to manage it on a daily basis.*

It can be exceptionally easy to get caught up in the drama of wanting to lose weight – to find excuses and reasons why our diet and exercise plan has not come together – but if we take a step back and consider what we really need to look at to get our lives on track, it comes down to optimising our energy levels. When we feel good and have the energy to get through the entire day, along with the ever-increasing demands and expectations each new day presents, life becomes a whole lot easier. We are able to deal with any unexpected stress, manage our time more efficiently, and be organised enough to eat well and finish each day feeling satisfied and in control, rather than exhausted and dreading the next one.

The funny thing about energy is that while we often look outside ourselves to seek it via pills, caffeine, stimulants or external motivators, much of our ability to generate, maintain, control and manage our energy levels comes from our own ability to retreat within and learn to understand our minds and bodies and what they need at any particular time to be at their best. At various points in time this may equate to eating certain types of food, at others taking rest and relaxation or regular physical activity to recharge and reignite a body that is used to sitting in an air-conditioned office for 10 hours each day.

When we are feeling tired and overwhelmed, the first thing we can do to get back on track is to remember the basic energy laws. This will always be the starting point to making the various lifestyle changes that we need to take charge of in order to get back in control of our own energy level and life.

The laws of optimal energy

MANAGE YOUR FUEL INTAKE

Busy people are notorious for forgetting how important it is to eat well-balanced meals and snacks regularly throughout their long working day. It is common to see a businessman or busy part-time mum skip breakfast in favour of coffee and then not eat again until 2 or 3 in the afternoon. Is it any wonder why we fail to be at our best when we have no good-quality fuel in our systems to cope with the demands of life? Your body is a machine, a finely tuned one that cannot run on empty and yet we expected it to day after day, year after year.

The crucial aspect of eating for optimal energy is keeping your blood glucose levels as stable as possible. Low blood glucose levels can make you feel tired, hungry and even irritable, and levels drop when balanced amounts of carbohydrates and proteins are not consumed regularly throughout the day. Aiming to have small, frequent meals and mid meals every 3–4 hours is all you need to do to achieve optimal blood glucose control. Ideally, this fits into a pattern of eating breakfast, morning tea, lunch, afternoon tea and dinner. Always choose one food that contains low-glycaemic index carbs, such as grain bread or crackers, low-fat dairy, fruit or wholegrain cereal, with one protein-rich food such as low-fat dairy, lean meat or nuts. Food examples that achieve this balance include crackers and cheese, yoghurt and fruit, grain bread with lean tuna or ham, or oats and milk.

The second dietary area to work on when it comes to maintaining optimal energy levels is to make sure that you are eating energy nutrient-rich foods that contain the key vitamins and minerals that are involved in energy production. The B group vitamins – iron, zinc and iodine – are just some of the key nutrients we need on a daily basis to ensure our body can access our stored fuel efficiently. Aiming to include lean red meat in your diet at least 3–4 times each week, eating oily fish at least twice each week, along with wholegrain breads and cereals and brightly coloured fresh fruits and vegetables in large quantities every day, will help you ensure that you tick all these nutritional boxes.

WATCH THE STIMULANTS

Stimulants, in particular caffeine consumed in energy drinks, tea, coffee or diet soft drinks, can be a major issue when it comes to aiming for constant, sustained energy levels throughout the working day. While a stimulant will give you a sudden hit of energy, the lull that follows can make you feel even more tired and lethargic than you did before. For this reason, controlling your intake of stimulant drinks and caffeine is crucial if your goal is to optimise your energy levels throughout the entire day at work. Sure, there is nothing wrong with enjoying a coffee a day, but working towards drinking more water and herbal tea will be a habit that serves your energy levels well long term.

SCHEDULE YOUR EXERCISE

When you are feeling tired, run-down and overweight, exercise is the first thing to go, while in fact it should be the first thing you focus on to feel better. When you increase your heart rate, and blood is sent pumping through your body, miraculous things happen. Suddenly your cells' energy centres are firing, more air fills your lungs and the body awakens. This is why you always feel better after you have done some exercise. We know that exercise is good for us in general, but perhaps even more so for individuals who spend considerable amounts of time sitting down. It is known that many hours of sitting slows down a number of important metabolic processes, and basically our metabolic rate long term. The slower our metabolism runs, the more tired and sluggish we feel, and for those of us who need to be at our best cognitively and physically, this means that regular exercise must be a focal point in our week, no matter how busy we are.

MOVE YOUR BODY

While exercise that significantly increases heart rate is important, so too is the simple act of moving around each day. Making an effort to get out of the office at lunchtime, walking up and down stairs, and walking to work are simple daily additions that go a long way in restoring the body's natural cycles and moving the body the way it is programmed to be each and every day. It can be as simple as setting the timer on your computer to remind you to get up every hour, or making sure that you enjoy lunch away from your desk, but it is an imperative focus for individuals who spend much of their working day sitting in an office environment.

GET SOME SUNLIGHT

As a result of living a modern, busy life it is common to see adults with low vitamin D levels, simply because we do not get outside into the sunshine. The issue with vitamin D when it comes to energy levels, mood and performance is that a low level of this vitamin makes you feel as if you have been run over by a bus. This feeling, when combined with a poor diet and limited exercise, is a sure-fire way to ensure that you are feeling below par each and every day. And unlike other nutrient deficiencies for which the standard therapy is a vitamin supplement, the best way you can make sure that your vitamin D level is topped up is to spend some time outdoors each day. Not only is getting some fresh air each day good for your health in general, it also contributes to keeping your vitamin D at the right level so that your body's energy levels can be naturally regulated.

PRIORITISE SLEEP

Sleep is a little like food when it comes to energy levels. We know getting enough sleep will help us feel better, and control our cravings, appetite and weight, and yet we continually make the decision to get far less sleep than we need to be at our best. Whether these situations evolve because we fall asleep in front of the television, spend too much time out socialising or because we are so wired after a day filled with stress and stimulation is irrelevant; all we need to know is that 5–6 hours' sleep each night is not enough. If your ultimate goal is to feel better, optimise your energy levels and get your body and weight under control, you need to commit to getting at least 7 hours' sleep each night during the first half of the week – without exception.

LEARN TO TAKE A MENTAL BREAK

Whether your mental break is 5–10 minutes each hour, an exercise class at lunchtime, a power nap or a meditation break each afternoon, the demands of technology, long working days and constant access to email and social media mean that we need to learn to give our minds a break. It is common for us to wake up in the morning and check our emails, be online for 12–14 hours a day, sit in front of the television for another 2–3 hours and then go to bed playing with our phones.

The brain does not cope well with this constant stimulation; it needs time to think freely, switch off, consolidate and relax. Too often, we fail to give it this time. What results is restlessness, an inability to concentrate and think clearly, insomnia, irritability, a lowered immune system, poor quality sleep and a general feeling of fatigue. While each and every one of us will have a different method of taking a mental break, particularly at times when we recognise these symptoms are negatively impacting our energy levels, it is time to regroup and consider ways in which we can add regular mental breaks in our life on a daily basis.

TECHNOLOGY-FREE TIME

Heaven forbid this should even be suggested out loud: take a complete break from technology. This means no mobile phone, no internet and no social media, including television, to give your mind a complete break from external stimulation to let it go within and think freely. Ideally, this can be an action that is implemented on a daily basis, so you can have a couple of hours each day to return to a more simple way of being, and the pleasures and joys of life that come with that.

QUALITY RELATIONSHIP TIME

If one thing has been proven to suffer in modern life, it is the quality of our relationships. Divorce and marital breakdowns are common, we acknowledge that we do not spend enough time with those closest to us, and relationships are brief, superficial and lack meaning. One of the most important aspects of being human is the ability to form meaningful relationships with others, whether it is with work colleagues, other mums at school or our intimate partners. And building and maintaining these relationships needs time. To be able to give relationships this time in today's frantic world, we need to allocate time. Each and every workday, and each and every weekend, our most precious relationships need time allocated to them in which they can build, regenerate and flourish long term.

TIME TO RELAX AND REGROUP

Relationships need time and none more so than the relationship we have with ourselves. Time spent alone to think, process, make decisions and nurture the self. Sadly this is the time that is most often shifted to other areas of our lives, whether it be to our partners, our work, our kids or other commitments. The first step you can take towards making this time is to become aware of how little time you currently spend on time for the self, and then work towards creating time, even if it is just an hour or two each month, in which you can fully be you without distraction, pressure or expectation.

The Monday to Friday rules

❁ *Rules give human beings structures and guidelines
to help them make numerous decisions on a daily
basis.*

Human beings need rules. We need them simply because when
we are left to our own devices we tend to push limits. In real life
we stay too long in parking places, forget to give way to others
when driving and need to be told that we cannot drink and drive.
When it comes to food, as we live in a time in which high-fat,
high-calorie food is far too readily available, only the most self-
regulated among us manage to control ourselves on a daily basis
and not overeat. For this reason, developing some of your own
food rules is a good way to learn to manage your food intake
behaviour and know what your personal limits need to be. For
some of us this will translate into being strict with ourselves 80%
or 90% of the time, while for others it may mean training at high
intensity numerous times throughout the week to compensate for
eating a lot. While each of us will feel comfortable with a different
set of food rules, here are some extremely useful ones that form the
basis of the Monday to Friday Diet.

No alcohol during the week

Alcohol tends to slip into our lives gradually and before we know
it, we are drinking on most nights of the week. The issues with
this are that alcohol is high in calories, we tend to eat more when
we are drinking, and we drink at a time of the day when we are

particularly sedentary and hence do not burn the alcohol calories off. Choosing to go 'alcohol-free' at least for the first four days of the working week is a good way to balance your lifestyle, calorie intake and weight, and is a rule that will serve you well throughout your life.

One low-calorie day

People like diets because a 'diet' gives them an opportunity to reset, refocus and reboot – in other words, a chance to completely focus on eating nothing but nutritious, low-calorie food and reap the benefits of doing so, even after just a day or two. One of the issues with modern life is that we rarely get the time or opportunity to achieve a good balance between eating out, being social and maintaining a controlled dietary intake to ensure weight control. Setting aside a day each week in which you significantly lower your calorie intake and focus on eating only unprocessed, low-calorie fresh fruits and vegetables is a great habit to build so that each week you remind yourself of how much fresh food you need on a daily basis to be at your best. Alternating the number of calories you eat throughout the week is also known to be a useful strategy to constantly challenge your metabolic rate, with the goal of making your cells burn fat as efficiently as possible.

'Must train' days

This is where the mantra 'no excuses' needs to kick in. Too often we miss training sessions when we simply cannot afford to. Staying on top of our weight in a world in which we are less and less active but have easy access to more and more calories means we must have a minimum number of training sessions we commit to each week and stick to this commitment, no matter what. Something always happens and there is always an excuse, but the harsh truth is that there are people who manage to get their training done no matter what, and then there are those who have excuses. This does not mean that you have to train every single day, nor does it mean you have to commit to an expensive trainer to achieve the results you are looking for. It simply means that if you really want to keep on top of your weight, you will have to commit to a minimum number of good quality training sessions every single week.

Bring lunch to work 4 days a week

If you could calculate how much money you have spent buying your lunch over the past 10 years, chances are that you could have afforded a trip to an island paradise for a week with the money. Not only is buying your lunch at work an expensive luxury, rarely do the lunch selections found within food courts tick the nutritional boxes we need them to.

Making a commitment to bring your lunch to work at least 4 days every week has numerous benefits. First, it means you have complete control over your food selections and hence can ensure that you have the right nutritional balance that will support your weight-loss goals. Second, it means you can ensure that you have the 2–3 cups of salad or vegetables you need to keep full, as well as the right amount of carbohydrates from a small amount of bread, rice, crackers or beans. And third, it means that you will be organised and have your supplies on hand to make a nutritionally balanced lunch that will ultimately save you a lot of money.

The key to finding time to prepare your lunches is to make them the night before. Rarely do we have time in the morning to be able to put together a well-balanced lunch, which means that planning ahead is the key. Perhaps try to make an extra meal a week that can be used for lunches, know what you need to throw together quickly to get the right mix of proteins, carbs and vegetables, or schedule a trip to the supermarket each Sunday or Monday at lunchtime to stock up for the week ahead. While it may seem a little boring, keeping a tight control of your calories for at least half the week will help keep your calories down for most of the week and your diet on track.

No treats until Friday

Treats are another food area that we need rules for. The abundance of cakes, biscuits, chocolates, lollies and other treats means that without rules we run the risk of eating these high-calorie foods multiple times every day. If you are blessed with an amazing metabolism you may be able to enjoy these treats often but for most of us, particularly those who are office bound, we simply do not burn enough calories.

While there may be a few tough souls who can say yes to just one biscuit or a thin slice of cake, the more commonly observed human behaviour is the scenario in which we find it hard to say no and have polished off 4 or 5 biscuits, or 3 chocolate brownies, simply because they were left in front of us at work. For this reason, having a clearly defined rule in your head that makes the commitment of no treats until Friday will make your food decisions a whole lot easier to make.

Compensate when you have overdone things

When you do find that you have eaten something that perhaps you should not have, or when you have had a big function or meal out, one of the most important Monday to Friday Diet rules to learn is to compensate when you have overdone things. This might mean simply cutting back a little and being strict with your calorie intake for your next meal, or it could also mean scheduling in an extra training session or walk. But this rule gets you into a powerful lifelong habit of compensating when you have eaten a little too much, as we all do at times, simply because we are human.

One coffee a day

If there is one weekday habit that is the undoing of many a diet, it is our increasing reliance on coffee to get through the day. Whether it is a flat white, macchiato or caramel latte, endless coffees with added milk and sugar represent a disaster when it comes to weight control. Not only do the stimulatory effects of caffeine play with your body's natural hunger and satiety signals, but the extra calories in the milk and other additions are not adequately compensated for, which basically means we are drinking more and more calories without lowering our food intake.

While there is nothing wrong with coffee, and a cup or two a day may actually have powerful health benefits, the issue lies in relying on multiple cups of milk-based coffee to get through your day. For this reason, having a strict limit of one milk-based coffee each day will go a long way when it comes to controlling your calorie intake and weight control long term.

Time out for self every day

It is exceptionally easy to get so caught up in the day-to-day frenzy of life that we forget the basic things that we need to do in order to keep our heads clear and our lives on track. Simply committing time, even just a few minutes every day, to regroup, refocus and clarify what you want to get done will allow you to self-manage stress and time and keep your personal needs and boundaries at the forefront of your mind. You can start with as little as 5 minutes a day, allocated to free thought and meditation, and ideally this will be scheduled in at a similar time each day so it becomes a habit. Long term, your mental health is likely to benefit with as much as an hour allocated to this purpose a day.

No excuses

If there is one difference between those who achieve what they set out to do and those who never quite get there, it is that achievers do not accept excuses. When road humps pop up or when things do not quite go to plan, achievers push on and find other ways to get things done.

There are two reasons why excuses rear their ugly heads in life – first, because we do not want to do what we have said we need to do to get where we want to go, or second, because we can have a tendency to be slack and lazy. Once you work out which of these is the underlying reason for your excuse, you can then work out the best way to move forward. In the case of not wanting to do what you need to, there is always the option of choosing another way to get where you want to go. For example, in the case of weight loss, a different diet or type of exercise might be the solution. When it comes to being slack and lazy, this simply requires a reality check, and sometimes we need to be told that our behaviour is 'below the line' and it is time to step it up.

The Monday to Friday principles

Know the difference between weekdays and weekends

For many of us, there is little difference between our social commitments during the week and on the weekend. We have functions and events to attend on most nights of the week and there is little to no time left to relax and do nothing. When it comes to our diets and training regime, this then tends to mean that higher calorie, high-fat eating slips in to many of our weekdays as it does the weekends, and training/exercise sessions can be readily dropped in favour of a 'better offer'.

In order for us to take control, we have to make a clear distinction in our own lives between what we need to do on weekdays versus the weekends. It may mean that sometimes we need to stay home and cook rather than go out for dinner with friends, that we have to go to the gym even though our favourite TV program is on, and that we have to leave a function early so we can get to bed and, in turn, get up early enough the next day to prepare lunch and go to the gym. While each of us will have our individual weekday–weekend balance that works best for us, taking control may still mean that sometimes we need to pull back in the week in order to keep our health and weight-loss goals on track.

Start your weekdays early

Starting the day early has several benefits for the metabolism. It also means that you have more time in the morning to train, eat breakfast and arrive at work with plenty of time to get organised and stuck into your work before everyone else arrives. You have time to pack your lunch, walk to work and plan your day, and you feel more in control. When you feel in control you are far more likely to keep on track with your goals.

There is no secret to getting up early; it is something that we basically have to train ourselves to do. While there is no doubt that some of us are 'morning people', ultimately, in a busy working world, those who get ahead are the ones who also tend to start the day early. When you choose to train in the morning, your session is out of the way for the day and your metabolism is up and running. Eating your breakfast early will help you burn more calories throughout the day, and starting your work day early will ensure you get more done and can leave the office in time for training, dinner or much needed down time.

If you are one of those souls who have every good intention of getting out of bed earlier but then hit the snooze button 20 times, you are thinking about it too much. The best way to break this habit is to get out of bed as soon as the alarm goes off – the more you think about it, the less likely you are to get up. Then try to create a morning ritual that helps the morning become an enjoyable part of your day as opposed to a dreaded reality. Program your phone to play your favourite tunes when you wake up, read something inspirational, brew your favourite coffee or do some stretches. Easing into the day rather than rushing is the ideal way in which we should embrace and greet every new day.

Shift your mindset from resentment to opportunity

Many people live their lives constantly counting down to the weekend. While we may not always love our jobs and would much rather be at home than working, having such a strong dislike for work sets us up for a pretty miserable existence. This mindset means that we are approaching the working week to 'get through' rather than 'live' and inevitably much unhappiness can stem from this.

If you hate your job and are constantly counting down the days and hours until your next weekend or vacation, it may be time to work on shifting your mindset. If we approach things we do not like with a negative mindset, we tend to spiral our thoughts downwards into more and more negativity, which can leave us feeling worse and worse. If, instead, we seek to identify what our work does offer us, and the way in which it actually helps our life, our working week will start to look brighter.

Spend some time considering what your job or role offers you, even if the only benefit is your income. Then use this energy to consider the ways in which you could use your position to benefit you. Could you change your hours, or use your breaks to focus on personal programs or on your health and fitness? What other job opportunities are there available, and if you are really that miserable, is it worth considering a job change? One thing is certain, if you really despise your job or working environment that much, the only person really, really suffering is you, so perhaps it is time to break free.

Work towards weekday balance

Working towards weekday balance means that no matter how many hours you work each day, or how busy you are, you always factor some nice things into your day. This may be having a coffee or lunch with a friend, scheduling a workout or chatting on the phone. Without these simple daily pleasures it can be exceptionally easy to get caught up in the day-to-day grind and forget how to enjoy the small things in your day. Start by working towards one nice thing that you do each day and look forward to, and then also start to plan your weeks this way. Once you have regular training, social and personally enjoyable experiences scheduled throughout your week, each and every week will be so much more appealing and ultimately enjoyable, work or no work.

Develop your own personal rules

While the Monday to Friday Diet can provide the food structure to help control your weight, every single person will need a slightly different approach depending on their age, gender, personal and family commitments, and lifestyle goals. Some people may like to be strict in the week and relax on weekends, and others may like to exercise once or twice a week only. Whatever your personal preference and interests are, developing a weekday structure that works for you and that you stick to, is the best step you can take to get your health and fitness under control.

Super Saturday

❁ *Weekdays are for working, Sundays for relaxing, and that only leaves Saturdays to set the platform for the week ahead.*

For some of us, Saturday means a sleep-in and a lazy brunch with friends; for others it is simply another workday, or an exceptionally busy day running around completing errands and taking kids to parties, sport and friends' houses. Whatever Saturday means to you, when it comes to getting your Monday to Friday Diet on track, Saturday means taking control, getting organised and seizing whatever time you can manage to find for yourself.

In today's busy world, it could be argued that being organised is the key to life success. Unfortunately, this seemingly simple concept is easier said than done, with busy professionals often struggling to find the time to actually get organised. In the same way that our approach to weekdays tends to predict our diet and exercise success, so too does the way we approach the limited free time that we have. Once upon a time our weekends were our time out – no work or commitments until Monday morning – a whole 48 hours to relax, regroup and zone out. Nowadays Saturday tends to look more like a standard weekday, with school sports, exercise classes and numerous other commitments that dominate our so-called 'free time'. Then this leaves Sunday, a single day, for us to relax and unwind. And while Sunday may seem a good day to get organised, perhaps Saturday is the better day simply because we are already in the buzz of doing rather than relaxing.

Getting organised on a Saturday does not have to mean hours spent cooking or shopping or preparing food. Rather, it simply means spending a few minutes considering what commitments you have for the week ahead, what basic groceries you will need in order to prepare some lunches and healthy dinners and, if you are super organised, a meal or two ready-made so you can really take Sunday off to spend as you would like.

Sacred Sunday

❀ *In a whirlwind existence, making a commitment to a*
Sacred Sunday – a day when you can regroup, refocus,
rest and spend quality time with those closest to you –
can be the difference between living and surviving.

Sunday can be the best day of the week, or the worst. It is traditionally the special day of rest for friends and family to come together and
be reminded of the simple things in life that bring us pleasure. More
often than not, however, Sunday becomes a frantic day of fitting in
as much as we can before another week rolls around – so it is not
surprising that many of us start the week feeling as if we need a break.

In order to take control of your Sunday, it is time to consider when
was the last time you enjoyed a whole day without any plans,
commitments or social events. When you could simply be at home,
in your space and do exactly what you wanted, when you wanted.
When you could sleep as long as you wanted to, have a little afternoon nap, potter, relax and simply be.

Chances are that you cannot remember the last time you did this –
hence the call for 'Sacred Sundays'. Allocate a Sunday, even just once
a month, in which you do absolutely nothing – treat it as a mini
break to re-centre and find yourself again in this frantic world, to
rest rather than do, to relax and see what happens rather than plan,
to just be.

Human beings need this time out. Prior to constant electronic
stimulation from the internet, mobile phones and television, extra-
long working hours, kids' sport and errands becoming the focus of
the weekend, families regularly had this time, whether it was in the

hours after an evening mealtime of 6pm or on Saturday and Sunday. Time to think, to dream, to talk to loved ones and pay attention to the small things in life that bring us the most pleasure, whether it be the conversation over a family meal at the table, playing a game in the backyard or going for a walk around the neighbourhood together. Studies have repeatedly shown that the simple act of eating a family meal together on four occasions each week sees children grow up with lower body weights, better psychosocial functioning and a lower rate of mood disorders.

For Type A-multi-taskers, the thought of committing to regular weekend downtime without plans or commitments can seem extremely daunting, but if you consider the intense demands we place on ourselves, our time and our relationships, it becomes easier to see that an annual holiday or occasional 3-day weekend does not allow adequate time throughout the year to achieve a good balance between work, play and unplanned rest. To regain control over our own lives and achieve this ever elusive balance, we have to actively schedule this time in, for the benefit of our health and our soul.

Perhaps most importantly, the introduction of 'Sacred Sundays' allows much needed time to nurture our relationships with ourselves and those closest to us. Sacred Sundays also present a perfect opportunity to foster some of your own family- or friend-based rituals – rituals such as Sunday lunch that start to become more of a focus in your life and which also help to bring much meaning to special times spent together, which in turn nurtures the relationships which fight to survive in busy modern life.

When it comes to our diet and exercise regimens, while Sunday is not the day for strict gym sessions and gym regimens, it is a time to concentrate on good quality food, ensuring you are ready for the week ahead, and moving your body as much as you can.

The weekend challenge

❖ *As long as I eat well during the week, can I have weekends off?*

What to eat on weekends

What is it about the weekend that regularly sees a week of relatively well-controlled eating quickly replaced with 48 hours of continual eating and drinking and often completely overindulging until Monday morning, under the proviso that it is 'the weekend'. While there is nothing wrong with enjoying your weekend with plenty of good food, wine and company, a weekly habit of consuming many, many more calories than anyone needs simply because it is the weekend is a habit that has to be broken.

Weekends can present a whole new range of challenges when it comes to our diet, exercise and weight control. Many social occasions are food focused, so we are more likely to drink alcohol and eat out, while psychologically the weekend tends to be time to relax and let things go a little, eating things we usually would not and skipping exercise altogether. Unfortunately, modern life tends to be so indulgent that few of us are able to do this and still achieve good weight-loss results. For this reason we need to consider the key aspects of the weekend that impact our food and exercise regimens and brainstorm ways we can make sure these situations do not end up working against our weight-loss goals.

Whether it is programming imprinted in our brain when we are small, or because we are overly restrictive with our diets during the week and feel that we need to reward ourselves on weekends, straying too far from our calorie-controlled meal plans is a recipe for disaster – and research has proved this. The US Weight Control Registry, a research group that tracks the progress of people who have lost significant amounts of weight and kept it off for longer than 5 years, has shown that people who control their weight keep their food intake stable *most* of the time. What this means in relation to the weekend is that while they may enjoy a meal with more calories on special weekend occasions, this does not equate to an additional two milk-based coffees a day, a bottle of wine on Friday and Saturday nights as well as Sunday afternoon, and some extra cake with coffee as well as dessert simply because it is the weekend.

An observation is that we get things wrong on the weekend due to three main factors: too much alcohol, cafe-style eating and high-calorie restaurant or takeaway meals. These extra calories, combined with far less physical activity, mean that you can easily gain a kilo or two over the weekend and find yourself starting each week behind the eight ball when it comes to control-ling your weight. The good news is that just a few simple tricks will help you to balance your caloric intake over the weekend to ensure you can still enjoy your weekend minus the extra few kilos to match.

Cafe breakfasts

Eating brunch at your favourite cafe or restaurant is a lovely way to enjoy the weekend with friends and family, but heavy banana breads, Turkish toasts, large juices, pancakes and jumbo coffees contain far too many calories for the average person. Instead, focus on your protein-rich options of eggs, ricotta, smoked salmon or perhaps lean bacon, and aim for just one slice of grain or sourdough toast to balance the calories. Remember your mantra of 'no one needs a large coffee' and keep the freshly baked goods for special occasions only. Order extra vegetables such as mushrooms, spinach and tomatoes to give your cafe brekkie plenty of bulk, and keep in mind that you are unlikely to need to snack if your breakfast is much larger than it usually would be.

Cafe calorie counter

	CAL	CARBS (G)	FAT (G)
Eggs Benedict	1000	45	70
Pancakes	1000	175	25
Banana bread	300	60	18
Large smoothie	340	60	5
Large coffee	250	20	10
Eggs and bacon	600	30	50
Croissant	250	25	15
Bircher muesli	250	60	10
Egg and bacon roll	500	60	20
Ham and cheese omelette	300	10	20

Alcohol

When it comes to alcohol, self-control is the key. A highly controlled intake of wine and beer during the week is pointless if you then down 2–3 bottles of wine or 10–15 beers in a sitting over the weekend. Try to shift this binge drinking mentality to a more moderate approach in which you can enjoy a few alcoholic drinks without feeling the need to drink for the sake of it. Be mindful of spending time socially with people who encourage binge drinking, and whether you can limit heavier drinking occasions to just once or twice each week. Alcohol tends to be a habit rather than an enjoyable addition to life and for this reason can be managed.

Saturday night drinks

	CAL	CARBS (G)	SUGARS (G)
Bottle of beer (375ml)	135	7.5	0.8
Bottle of light beer	50	4.6	0.2
Schooner of beer	160	9.0	0.9
Glass of champagne	85	2.0	2.0
Glass of wine	80	0.2	0.2
Bottle of wine	525	3.8	3.8
Spirit with soda	70	0	0
Spirit with cola	120	7.5	7.5
Pre-mixed drink	230	33.8	33.3
Nip of liquor	45	3.8	3.8

Restaurant meals

The average fast food or restaurant meal will have at least 200 calories more than a meal you prepare for yourself at home simply because of the extra sauces, breads, oil and dressings and larger serving sizes. Have a substantial protein- or vegetable-based snack an hour or two before you venture out so you do not put a food order in while you are starving. Share meals where possible, especially dessert as portion sizes tend to be large, and again, try to

Saturday night meals

	CAL	CARBS (G)	FAT (G)
Pad Thai	420	33.1	22.8
Mushroom risotto	410	57.9	9.2
Hamburger and chips	900	97.9	43.3
Schnitzel and chips	720	40.7	35.1
3 slices thick pizza	675	99.0	28.9
Rack of ribs	1500	23.4	113.8
Steak and mash	475	24.0	25.0
Spaghetti marinara	450	88.0	2.5
Yum cha	630	72.0	25.0
Thai takeaway	570	58.0	30.1

avoid overeating simply because you are out. Training yourself to not eat extra simply because you are 'going out for dinner' is a key way to enable you to enjoy eating out regularly without the associated weight gain.

At coffee

Coffee catch-up dates are another common weekend commitment and while a coffee is fine, the toast, cakes, slices and banana bread treats are not as great, particularly if you are also having meals out over the weekend. Limit the number of coffees you enjoy over catch-ups and eat before you go so that you are not tempted with the high-carb treats generally served at coffee shops.

Coffee and tea

	CAL	CARBS (G)	FAT (G)
Small skim cappuccino	70	10	0
Mug of skim cappuccino	130	20	1
Large regular latte	220	17	12
Piccolo latte	30	2	2
Regular hot chocolate	250	30	10
Regular caramel latte	280	36	10
Regular chai latte	330	40	14
Green tea	3	0	0
Long black	2	0	0
Skim iced coffee	165	30	0

At restaurants

It may surprise you to learn that eating out does not have to mean overeating – you simply need to be mindful of your choices and know how to get the right balance when ordering off a menu. The first rule when it comes to restaurant meals is to never go out for a meal starving or you will be sure to overeat. Look for light entree options of salad or seafood, or share an entree with your partner. When you are choosing main meals, think protein and vegetables such as steak, fish or chicken, and order extra sides of vegetables. Remember that grilled dishes always contain much less fat than fried or crumbed options, and always ask for dressings and sauces on the side, while avoiding cream-based meals entirely. Finally, if you really do feel like dessert, always share, as the most pleasure from dessert is experienced in the first couple of mouthfuls.

Family functions

Family events are notorious for seeing us regress into the eating habits of our youth. We will search for snacks we enjoyed as children even though we never eat them as adults, binge on foods with our parents and siblings and forget the food rules we have worked so hard to commit to in adulthood. For one-off special occasions this poses no major issue but if you find yourself at family functions weekly, you may need to work towards not regressing into the eating patterns of your youth. Remember your food rules and seek out plenty of vegetables and salad and enjoy a single dessert, not multiple serves simply because a well-meaning relative has made it for you.

The movies

What you choose to eat at the movies tends to also be a programmed response – if you always grab a choc-top or large popcorn, chances are that you will do it whether you are hungry or not. Work towards never going to the movies hungry and indulging in one small treat that you share rather than pretending that the calories do not count simply because you are eating them in the dark.

Movie food

	CAL	CARBS (G)	FAT (G)
Small popcorn	170	19	9
Large popcorn	540	60	30
Large soft drink	270	66	0
Choc-top	280	30	20
Large packet of potato chips	450	50	20
Large packet of chocolates	800	100	36
Nachos	600	60	60
Packet of jelly lollies	680	160	0

Aside from these tricks and tips for specific weekend eating occasions, another simple way of keeping your food intake under control is to follow as normal a food routine on the weekend as possible. If you do have breakfast or lunch out, compensate with a light soup or salad for the following meal. If you find that you have eaten a number of heavier meals over the weekend, have a lighter day or two of eating early in the week. We live in a world of constant calorie overloading and minimal activity and for this reason we cannot wipe out two days of the week if we want to maintain, let alone lose weight, so identify your food rules and stick to them, even on the weekends.

Reset Monday

❂ *The way you begin your week is the way you will live your week.*

The way we begin our week is a powerful indicator of the way we will live our week. Monday offers us hope, excitement and opportunity. It is the day when we get a fresh start; the time of the week when our good health and fitness intentions can be used to our advantage if and how we know the right way to implement healthy lifestyle changes and maintain them. A well-organised and planned

Monday can ultimately mean that 3–4 days of our week are on track. And when you translate that into your caloric intake, meal planning and exercise sessions, 3–4 good days ultimately means weight loss over the course of a week.

Unfortunately for many of us, Monday mornings start in a rushed and frazzled state where we are happy to have simply made it to work, as opposed to starting the week fresh and organised to help us keep on track with our diet and weight-loss goals. If you adhere to the mantra 'the way you start your day is the way you live your day', then there is much to be gained from making a concerted effort to start each Monday on the right foot, especially when it comes to having your food and exercise plans ready to help you stay focused and make positive progress.

A good Monday will begin beautifully – this means sitting down and enjoying breakfast; taking time out to plan the week ahead and outline what you are keen to achieve; and being grateful that you are here at all to enjoy a brand-new week. For some of us this may come naturally with a new week signalling a new start, but others may need to do some work to learn to appreciate Mondays rather than hate them.

If you consider that Monday is an opportunity to reboot, recharge and kick-start your week after the weekend, this is a great way to take control of your diet again. There is evidence to show that including a low-calorie food day as part of your overall calorie intake will give the metabolism a boost and compensate when things have gone off track over the weekend. Knowing that Monday has been reserved for light foods and low-calorie eating will help to get rid of the extra fluid and bloating that accompanies a weekend filled with alcohol and high-fat, high-salt foods. Eating lightly reminds us of how good we feel when we get back in touch with our hunger and satiety signals, and it also helps us to drop the couple of kilos that tend to be gained over a weekend filled with social engagements.

Training Tuesday

❖ *Mondays are the day to recover after the weekend,*
  Tuesdays are to get serious.

Tuesday is traditionally the action day of the week when things really get moving, with meetings planned, appointments booked and serious projects underway. Tuesday is also a big day for exercise – visit any gym on a Tuesday night and you will be sure to find it packed with members who are working off the sins of the weekend. For this reason, Tuesday is the best day of the week to get serious when it comes to your diet and exercise regimen. It is early enough in the week to get some real results when it comes to training and weight loss and it also gives you enough time to establish momentum before the weekend rolls around again.

Unlike Reset Monday, in which calorie intake is significantly reduced to help give you a weight-loss kick-start at the beginning of the week, Tuesday should focus on calorie-controlled, high-protein eating that you can maintain for the next few days. The emphasis is on nutrient-dense eating and a good balance between your carbo-hydrate and protein intake so you feel full and satisfied throughout the day and less tempted by extra snacks and high-calorie treats. Tuesday is a good day to stay at home after work and prepare both physically and psychologically for the rest of the week. While this may mean saying no to social engagements, it will also mean that you have built a platform from which you can keep on track easily for the remainder of the week.

When it comes to exercise, on Tuesday things get a little more serious. Many of us find ourselves constantly pressed for time, so when we do schedule time for training we need to go hard. Long gone are the days when a walk is enough; if we are to really take control of our weight and give our metabolism a much needed boost, when we do find time to workout we have to make sure we are actually training our muslces to burn calories more efficiently, not simply to maintain our current weight. To achieve this, the programs or classes we choose or the type of cardio sessions we attend need to be monitored with clear targets to make sure we are burning as many calories as we can in the precious time we are able to allocate to exercise.

Humpday Wednesday

❁ *The way you view and spend your Wednesdays will make or break your weekday commitment.*

Wednesday means progress, hard work and focus. It means learning to juggle work, exercise and social demands while keeping a strong focus on your health and fitness goals. Unfortunately, Wednesday is when things can start to go off track – the demands of the week begin to ramp up, social engagements are scheduled, you start to get tired and the end of the week is in sight. Taking control of what you eat and do on Wednesday is a crucial component of your Monday to Friday Diet. If you go off track on a Wednesday, the chances that you will be gaining weight rather than losing it are high.

For many of us, while we may begin each week with a set of clear goals and plan of attack, by Wednesday interruptions and unforeseen events mean that it tends to be Wednesday when things can start to go off track. For this reason, Wednesday, the halfway point in our working week, is the day to take some time out and take stock of the way the week has been progressing.

Wednesday means allocating some time during the day to consider what social engagements are looming over the weekend and what potential impact this will have on your food intake. Take time to consider if you are on track with your exercise goals for the week and, if not, schedule sessions throughout the remaining days of the week.

When it comes to weight loss, Wednesday needs to focus on a tightly controlled calorie intake and a short but intense training session. This balance is particularly important if you regularly eat out on a Wednesday because you need to compensate for a higher caloric intake at dinner. Additionally, dining out also means that consideration needs to be given to restaurant choices. Whether this means knowing what to eat at a breakfast meeting, work conference or quick dinner before a date, because each and every food decision adds up throughout the course of a week, being mindful of which food choices will best serve your diet goals is a crucial part of keeping on track. While a common way of approaching meals enjoyed away from home is to throw all self-imposed dietary limits and rules out the window, Wednesday is too early in the week to do this if your ultimate goal is weight loss.

In exercise language, as time becomes more and more precious as the week rolls on, Wednesday means quality over quantity when it comes to your choice of exercise. Sure, if you can spare an hour or two to walk and exercise by all means schedule it in. But if you struggle to find this time, then commit to a short, intense 20–30-minute session each Wednesday to not only help give your metabolic rate a quick boost but to allow plenty of other time in your day to work, plan and play.

Funday Thursday

❉ *For some people, Thursday is their favourite day of the week; for others it's their least.*

Thursday can drag on if you have managed to negotiate Friday off, or go like a flash in situations where companies try to get as much done as they can before the end of the week. Food-wise, Thursday can be extremely challenging, as this is the day when work lunches and outings are common and, as social commitments increase, it can become more and more difficult to control your calorie intake. In addition to this, fitting in training sessions also becomes more challenging, because as the second half of the week comes around we start to get tired and lose our motivation to go to the gym. Despite these challenges, Thursday can be a great day to strike a balance between the limitations of the working week and the opportunities of the upcoming weekend. All you need is a little structure on a Thursday, particularly during the first half of the day, and before you know it, you have made it to the end of the week with your weight-loss goals on track.

In terms of calorie intake, if you have remained focused from Monday to Wednesday, with Reset Monday and a big Training Tuesday, there will be some extra calories to play with by the time Thursday rolls around. Unfortunately, the extra calories in real terms means an extra 200–300 calories a day, or half a dessert in food terms, when the reality is that many of us consume an extra 500–600 calories in a sitting when we do let ourselves indulge. For this reason, if you find yourself socialising on a Thursday, a crucial skill to develop is the art of calorie compensation.

Calorie compensation means learning how much less you need to eat during the day to compensate for the extra calories you are planning to eat later. It also means learning how much extra movement and exercise you will need to factor in to negate any sins of a good meal or night out. For this reason, as Thursday will often be a day in which extra food calories are consumed, it is also one of the best days to book in a training session. Whether it is a personal training session with a trainer, a regular gym class or a social exercise session with a friend, a scheduled training session each Thursday is the best way to keep your exercise on track before the weekend.

TGI Friday

❉ *Once you have made it through the working week, surely you need a little reward?*

In an ideal world, no one would have to work on Fridays – we would be a lot more productive earlier in the week and Fridays would be the start of a standard 3-day weekend in which we could really relax and unwind. In modern life, however, Friday is an odd day at work. Lots of people take time off so the office is quieter, but for big businesses Friday is a working day just like any other, even though your mind may think otherwise. Friday is also the day when we like to let loose a little. There are often lunches and work drinks, and the relief of simply making it through another tough week can be licence enough to throw caution to the wind and eat and drink whatever we like. Luckily, all we need to know is how we can balance a little fun with our food and drink choices so we do not throw an entire week of hard work out the window.

Simply because it is Friday is not a reason to skip training – in fact, scheduling a session on a Friday is actually a good idea as it will help you to compensate for any extra calories that may have slipped in from extra alcohol and high-calorie food during the week. Plan your exercise session early in the day and support it with a light but filling breakfast. Once lunch and dinner come around, you will have a firm base from which to make reasonably healthy choices, even though your calorie intake may be higher than it usually is during the first half of the week.

Perhaps the next most important thing to consider on a Friday is who you spend your time with. Sure, there is nothing wrong with work drinks, but at the end of the day it is work and there is probably a lot to be said for enjoying a drink or two and then returning home to enjoy a good quality meal with those closest to you. The drinking culture of families, friendship groups and workplaces can be deeply entrenched and, as such, Friday night drinks can become an institution. While it is OK to have a drink, in the case of workplaces that offer an unlimited bar tab for employees or that provide large volumes of alcohol for staff members, the intention to drink as much as you can simply because it is free does need to be questioned.

A good way of managing Friday night drinks is to give yourself a predetermined limit and a curfew by which to go home and return to your real life. Establishing this before you get stuck into the wine will make it easier to know when it is time to stop, and also help you to maintain the boundaries between work and your personal life.

The Monday to Friday Diet

SUPER SATURDAY

The Saturday plan

1. Get organised.

2. Plan your meals.

3. Prepare before you go out.

4. Enjoy but do not overdo Saturday night.

5. Include some exercise.

❈ *The most powerful thing you can do to support your weight-loss goals is to allocate time each Saturday to get your food organised for the week ahead.*

Get organised

Chances are that you are already out and about on Saturdays and so it makes sense that you spend a few extra minutes stocking up on key supplies for the week ahead. Another benefit of stocking up for food supplies on Saturdays is that the fresh food in the stores is still fresh, whereas on Sundays the selection tends to be of far poorer quality.

Getting organised may mean completing your weekly shop or preparing some extra meals. It may mean ordering some meals online or cleaning out your cupboard or refrigerator. Whatever getting organised food-wise for the week ahead means to you, ultimately come Monday morning, little to no thought needs to go into what you will be eating on any given day, as it will already be planned out for you.

Your weekly staples shopping list

Wholegrain bread, wraps and crackers

Reduced-fat cheddar cheese

Cottage cheese

Goat's cheese/feta

Low-fat milk

Thick Greek-style yoghurt

Frozen berries

Frozen vegetables

Onions

Tomatoes

Mushrooms

Carrots

Lean mince

Eggs

Brown rice

Cans of tuna and salmon

Cans of beans

Reduced-salt stock

Tomato paste

Olive oil spray

Plan your meals

❖ *All you need to do is prepare one meal and a soup*
and you will have almost half the meals you need
for the week.

Simply by planning one or two meals as well as a soup each week, you will have almost half the meals you need for the week. Stir fries, casseroles, pasta bases and roasts can easily provide a couple of dinners as well as leftovers for lunch, and a big pot of soup will last an entire week whether it is used as a lunch base or as a quick dinner when you are in a rush. When you do find yourself with an hour or two to spare on a Saturday, instead of collapsing in front of the television, watch your favourite shows while you are quickly chopping and preparing a stir fry or casserole that can be frozen or cooked ready for the week ahead. For those professionals who work particularly long hours and find that they have dinner at work more often than not, home-prepared lunches are likely to be much more filling and nutritious than many of the options that are available close to workplaces.

The best meals to cook and freeze

Salmon Patties (page 86)

Hearty Dinner Soup (page 100)

Sesame Chicken (page 114)

Turkey Bolognaise (page 128)

Veggie Hot Pot (page 140)

✿ *The number one ingredient you can buy to help
ensure you eat well for the week ahead is salad – the
more salad you have, the better it will be for your
weight.*

Prepare before you go out

A common scenario come Saturday is that we spend the afternoon
running around finishing errands before again rushing out the door
for a Saturday night function or outing. Inevitably we have not
eaten particularly well during the day – only a coffee and perhaps a
lunch or breakfast out – and then we find ourselves ordering from
a menu when we are hungry and keen to enjoy a good meal. So,
rather than arriving at your favourite restaurant or pub starving and
ready to dive into the bread, chips and drinks, on Saturday afternoon factor in a filling, vegetable-rich snack before you head out.
Ideally, this snack should contain some protein and be consumed
one or two hours prior to going out to ensure that you are in control
of your hunger that night and more likely to make better choices
when dining out.

Saturday pre-party snacks

Meal replacement or protein shake

4 rye crackers with cottage cheese and tomato

Protein snack bar

½ cup natural yoghurt with ½ cup berries and 10 mixed nuts

Bowl of vegetable-based soup

❖ *A meal replacement shake is a specially formulated nutritional product that contains similar amounts of carbohydrates and proteins as a meal, with a much lower calorie content. Meal replacements are usually shakes or bars and can be used to replace a meal or as a filling snack choice to help prevent overeating. Look for products that contain 200 calories per serve, 20–30g of total carbohydrate and 15–20g of protein.*

A protein shake is usually a serve of 20–30g of concentrated milk protein that can be consumed with or without milk. Protein shakes are often used by athletes to help support muscle growth and recovery but can also be used as meal replacements or as high-protein snacks to help manage appetite between meals. When served with low-fat milk, a protein shake is not dissimilar to a meal replacement shake. Look for protein powders that contain 20–30g of protein per serve and less than 10g of total carbohydrate.

Enjoy but do not overdo Saturday night

❖ *There is a big difference between writing yourself off and enjoying a few drinks or a dinner out with friends.*

Saturday night is the night we tend to 'take off' – when we might indulge in a few drinks or eat a high-fat meal out. There is nothing wrong with this – in fact, it is absolutely imperative that we learn to balance social occasions as we cannot be a health and fitness purist all the time. Working towards this balance will simply require you to think of your Saturday outings as one-off occasions rather than writing off the entire weekend. If you are planning on having a big night, have a light lunch, or schedule in an extra training session to compensate. Learning to compensate will ultimately mean that you can enjoy your social occasions without negatively impacting your weight loss.

If you consider that a largish meal teamed with numerous alcoholic drinks can equate to more than 1000 calories in one sitting, being at least mindful of your food and alcohol choices, even though it is your 'night off', can be a powerful way to keep your weight under control and your head in the right space to be controlling your weight. This may mean swapping to a lower calorie alcoholic drink, or choosing your menu items carefully, but you will find that ditching the 'oh it doesn't matter, it's just one meal' mindset will help you to stay in control of your food intake in general.

Your best options when eating out

Grilled fish with a side serve of vegetables

Chicken cashew nut or prawn stir fry with ½ cup rice

Warm lamb or beef pumpkin salad

Sashimi with beans and vegetables

Grilled chicken or steak with vegetables

❀ *Love dessert on the weekends? In that case, always share desserts at a restaurant or cafe, and aim for just one heavy dessert each week, or choose a <100 calorie (400kJ) option after dinner.*

<100 calories (400kJ) desserts

1 small glass of wine

20g chocolate

1 scoop low-fat ice-cream

1 small dairy dessert

6 wafer crackers with 20g rich cheese

Include some exercise

❁ *Being busy is no longer an excuse; the secret to exercise is scheduling it in advance and committing to it each and every Saturday.*

Long gone are the days when we could take the weekend off; our weekdays are so busy that we simply have to make sure that we exercise on the weekends. It does not matter whether you go for a long walk with the family, meet a friend for a coffee and a walk, go to the gym or for a quick run before you head out on Saturday, as long as there is at least 30 minutes of some sort of activity that increases your heart rate every Saturday – no excuses.

❁ *Do you spend Saturdays taking the kids to and watching them at sport? This is the best time for you to do your exercise. Run or walk for even the first 20–30 minutes of the kids' sports activities and get your own exercise completed while they do theirs.*

Saturday exercise ideas

1. Start the day with a gym class or personal training session.

2. Meet a friend for a coffee and a walk.

3. Go for a walk or run while your kids are playing sport.

4. Walk to dinner or drinks rather than catching a cab.

5. Go for a late afternoon or early evening jog or walk.

❁ *What about snacks? To help control your calorie intake over the weekend, drop your snacks and stick to 3 meals a day, with an extra late-afternoon, low-calorie snack to help manage your appetite if you are planning to eat out.*

SATURDAY VEGETABLE TIP:
Before you head out to dinner, grab a carrot or cucumber and have a munch to take the edge off your hunger and boost your vitamin intake.

100-calorie snack choices

1 piece of fruit

Low-carb mini protein bar

1 slice low-fat cheese and two rye crackers

Carrot with 2 tbsp low-fat hummus

3 cups popcorn

Saturday meal plans

Breakfast
2-egg tomato, mushroom and spinach omelette OR Protein Pancakes (page 67). Small skim milk latte or flat white

Lunch
1 wholegrain wrap or 1 slice wholegrain bread toasted with 130g baked beans or small tin of tuna with ⅓ cup reduced-fat cheese, with 1–2 cups salad or bowl of vegetable-based soup

Dinner
Chilli Prawn Pasta (page 71) with 2 cups mixed salad and 1 small glass red or white wine

Breakfast
1 egg and 1 slice lean bacon on 2 slices grain bread with small skim milk coffee OR Breakfast Quesadillas (page 68)

Lunch
2 California sushi rolls and ½ cup (100g) fruit yoghurt OR Tuna Salad (page 70)

Dinner
Steak sandwich with 100g fillet steak on grain bread with 8 home-made sweet potato chips (100g) with tomato, lettuce and beetroot OR Low-Fat Chicken Curry (page 72)

Breakfast
Mushies on Toast (page 68) OR 1 slice sourdough toast with grilled mushrooms and sprinkled with 2 tbsp low-fat ricotta cheese with small skim coffee

Lunch

Stuffed Potato (page 70) or medium (150g) jacket potato topped with small can red salmon, ½ cup cottage cheese and chopped tomato, plus 1 apple, pear or orange OR Chicken Club Salad (page 69)

Dinner

Quick Chicken Pizza (page 71) with 2 cups mixed salad

Breakfast

Corn Fritters with Smoked Salmon (page 67)

Lunch

100g grilled lamb or chicken breast fillet with mixed salad greens and 100g sweet potato with 2 tbsp oil-free Caesar or ranch dressing OR Steak Wrap (page 69)

Dinner

Spicy Prawn Laksa (page 72) OR Thai Takeaway Stir Fry with prawns OR chicken & vegetables chicken cashew nut with ½ cup steamed rice

CORN FRITTERS WITH SMOKED SALMON

1½ cups corn kernels

1 egg

¼ cup plain flour

½ tsp bicarbonate of soda

¼ cup reduced-fat milk

2 tbsp chopped fresh parsley

1 tbsp extra-virgin olive oil

1 vine-ripened tomato, diced

½ avocado, diced

1½ cups baby spinach leaves

4 slices smoked salmon

1 In a small bowl place the corn, egg, flour, bicarbonate of soda, milk and parsley. Mix together with a fork to make a batter, crushing the corn a little. Season to taste with salt and pepper. Heat the olive oil in a frying pan over medium heat and cook the batter as 4 fritters (with about ⅓ cup of corn mix in each fritter) for 5 minutes on each side.

2 Place 2 fritters on a plate, then top with the tomato, avocado, spinach and salmon.

Serves 2

PROTEIN PANCAKES

1 egg

1 cup buttermilk

1 tbsp butter, softened

¾ cup plain flour

1 tsp baking powder

1 punnet berries

2 tbsp vanilla or berry protein powder

canola oil spray

ricotta cheese (optional)

1 Whisk egg, buttermilk and butter together. Stir in flour and baking powder. Add berries and protein powder.

2 Spray oil in frying pan and cook 2 tbsp batter over medium heat for 3 minutes, until pancake is brown, then turn over and cook for a further 2–3 minutes. Serve with a little ricotta cheese if desired.

Serves 4

MUSHIES ON TOAST

1 large or 4 small mushrooms

2 tsp olive oil

2 vine-ripened tomatoes

handful English spinach leaves

1 slice sourdough bread

20g feta cheese, crumbled

4 basil leaves, torn

1 Lightly sear mushrooms in a frying pan with olive oil. Add tomatoes and spinach and cook until tender. Toast bread.

2 Top toast with cooked vegetables and sprinkle with feta and basil.

Serves 1

BREAKFAST QUESADILLAS

1 egg and 1 egg white, beaten

¼ red onion, finely diced

½ red capsicum, finely diced

½ green capsicum, finely diced

1 slice lean ham or bacon

20g reduced-fat feta cheese

1 small wholemeal wrap

¼ avocado OR 1 tbsp extra-light sour cream

1 Scramble egg with onion and capsicum in a non-stick frying pan over medium heat.

2 Push to one side and lightly sear ham or bacon in the pan.

3 Crumble feta over egg mixture and wrap up with ham. Toast wrap.

4 Serve with avocado or sour cream.

Serves 1

STEAK WRAP

100g fillet steak, grilled and thinly sliced

2 tsp olive oil

1 brown onion, diced

1 tbsp brown sugar

2 slices beetroot

2 vine-ripened tomatoes

handful of rocket

1 small multigrain wrap

1 Sear steak with olive oil in hot frying pan for 7–10 minutes. Set aside.

2 Add onion, ¼ cup water and sugar and cook over medium heat until onion has softened and sugar has caramelised.

3 Pile steak, onions and salad on wrap.

Serves 1

CHICKEN CLUB SALAD

200g chicken breast fillet

50g 97% fat-free bacon

olive oil spray (optional)

4 vine-ripened tomatoes, sliced

½ small red onion, finely sliced

2 sticks celery, finely chopped

3–4 cups iceberg lettuce leaves

¼ cup reduced-fat mayonnaise

½ lemon, halved

1 Grill chicken breast until cooked. Slice and set aside.

2 Grill bacon or lightly fry with olive oil.

3 Slice bacon and mix with chicken and salad ingredients. Dress with mayonnaise and drizzle over lemon juice.

Serves 2

STUFFED POTATO

1 Pontiac potato

½ cup coleslaw with
low-fat dressing

1 roasted chicken breast,
finely sliced OR 100g cooked
lean chicken mince

2 tbsp creamed corn

1 Preheat oven to 210°C.

2 Pierce the potato a few times
and bake for 20–30 minutes,
until skin is crisp.

3 Combine coleslaw, chicken
and corn and spoon on top of
potato.

Serves 1

TUNA SALAD

100g green beans, trimmed

2 hard-boiled eggs, sliced
into quarters

2 x 95g cans tuna in spring
water, drained

1 small red onion, thinly
sliced

2 green onions, thinly sliced

250g cherry tomatoes, halved

100g mesclun lettuce

2 tsp finely grated
lemon rind

½ cup lemon juice

1 tbsp wholegrain mustard

2 gloves garlic, crushed

2 tsp sugar

1 Steam or microwave beans until
just tender. Cool and then halve
lengthways.

2 Combine beans with egg, tuna,
onions, tomato and lettuce in a
large bowl.

3 Whisk together remaining
ingredients in a small bowl;
add to salad and toss gently to
combine.

Serves 2

CHILLI PRAWN PASTA

14 cooked prawns

1 small zucchini, sliced and lightly cooked

1 roma tomato

2 cups of tomato pasta sauce

200g (1⅓ cups) fettucine

1 small chilli, finely sliced (optional)

2 or 3 olives (optional)

Heat prawns and vegetables in a little pasta sauce then mix through pasta. Add chilli and olives for a tasty lunch treat.

Serves 2

QUICK CHICKEN PIZZA

100g butternut pumpkin

100g chicken breast fillet

olive oil

2 onions, sliced

2 tbsp brown sugar

wholemeal Lebanese bread

2 tbsp tomato pasta sauce

1 cup baby spinach leaves

20g feta cheese, crumbled

1 Preheat oven to 200°C. Peel pumpkin and chop into 2cm cubes. Bake for 20–30 minutes, until tender.

2 Meanwhile, grill chicken or stir fry in 1 tsp olive oil.

3 Cook onion with 1 tsp oil over medium heat until translucent, add sugar and 2 tbsp water.

4 Top the Lebanese bread with pasta sauce and sliced chicken, onions, pumpkin, spinach leaves and feta. Lightly bake in the oven for 10 minutes until crispy. Serve with salad.

Serves 1

LOW-FAT CHICKEN CURRY

1kg chicken breast fillets, finely sliced

2 tbsp green curry paste

375g can reduced-fat coconut or evaporated milk

handful green beans

handful broccoli florets

½ red capsicum, sliced

227g can water chestnuts, drained

2 tbsp fish sauce

2 tbsp brown sugar

1 tbsp cornflour

1 cup cooked brown rice

1 Brown chicken in a little olive oil in a frying pan over medium heat, then add curry paste.

2 Add milk and bring to the boil, then reduce heat.

3 Add vegetables and simmer until lightly cooked.

4 Add fish sauce and sugar.

5 Mix cornflour with 2 tbsp water and add to mixture until curry thickens.

6 Serve with cooked brown rice.

Serves 4

SPICY PRAWN LAKSA

1 onion, finely chopped

1 tbsp green curry paste

1L salt-reduced vegetable stock

1 large carrot, finely sliced

1 red capsicum, sliced

1 small red chilli (optional)

40 green prawns

10 button mushrooms

375ml can light evaporated milk

⅓ cup cornflour

2 tbsp fish sauce

1 cup flat rice noodles

1 Cook onion in saucepan over medium heat until translucent. Add curry paste and cook until fragrant.

2 Add stock, carrot, capsicum and chilli (if using) and bring to the boil.

3 Add prawns and cook through.

4 Add mushrooms, milk, cornflour and fish sauce, and simmer for 10–15 minutes until cooked through.

5 Add noodles, cook for 4 minutes and serve into large bowls.

Serves 4

❀ Had a few drinks on Saturday night and not looking forward to waking up on Sunday? Have a sports drink or electrolyte solution before you crash to help prevent dehydration and hangovers.

SACRED SUNDAY

The Sunday plan

1. Be smart at brunch.

2. Commit to Sunday lunch.

3. Be active with friends or family.

4. Implement a technology ban.

5. Go light with your calories on Sunday night.

❀ It might alarm you to hear that your Sunday brunch may contain all the calories that you need for the entire day.

Be smart at brunch

If there is one day of the week in which we are more likely to enjoy a higher calorie breakfast, it tends to be Sunday. Whether this means having eggs and bacon at home or brunch at your favourite cafe, it also means that you can begin your Sunday with either a nutrient-rich, filling meal or a complete calorie overload. Now, while you may need a little extra fat at brekkie on Sunday, particularly if you have enjoyed a big night out on Saturday, you can still make some reasonably good choices at breakfast.

As a general rule of thumb, if you are including higher fat breakfast options such as eggs with cream, bacon or fried foods, limiting your bread intake by reducing the amount of toast you eat is a good way to compensate for those extra breakfast calories. Be mindful of liquid calories in juices, smoothies and large milk coffees, and if you do indulge in a largish breakfast, remember that your best option to control your calories for the rest of the day is to ditch lunch in favour of a light snack in the afternoon.

❀ *One slice of toast is equal to one regular milk coffee, so cut back if you tend to enjoy numerous milk coffees on Sundays.*

The best Sunday brunch choices

Poached eggs on toast

Vegetable omelette

Smoked salmon and ricotta with sourdough toast

Roasted tomatoes, mushrooms and spinach with egg or tofu

Bacon and egg sandwich on wholegrain toast

Commit to Sunday lunch

❀ *There is nothing more precious in life than enjoying good quality food with those closest to us on a regular basis.*

Our grandmothers and great-grandmothers spent all morning preparing Sunday lunch, and it, as well as the nap that followed afterwards, was, for many families, the entire focus of their weekly day of rest. The concept of Sunday lunch serves many different purposes. It brings families together and, as such, creates a certain level of respect and commitment for the family bond. It is also the perfect opportunity to commit to some healthy food preparation for the week ahead and creates an event in your week that brings people who care about each other together in a relaxed, calm way. Even if you can only commit to Sunday lunch once a month, it is a great tradition to begin with your family or even friends.

Whether you enjoy a roast dinner with lots of vegetables, a family BBQ or picnic-style meal, as long as your lunch choices include some vegetables and/or salad, you will not go wrong. Sunday lunches can also mean great lunch leftovers for Monday, and give way to a light meal on Sunday night to prepare for the week ahead.

❧ *There is research to support the coming together of families over meals throughout the week. Families who enjoy meals together over a table at least 3–4 times each week have teenagers who do better at school, are less likely to engage in drug and alcohol abuse and have higher ratings of psychosocial functioning.*

Be active with friends or family

Whether it is a walk, family cricket game, bushwalk or drive to the beach, Sunday is the perfect time for you to not only be active, but be active with those closest to you. For most of us it is a challenge to get the amount of exercise we require on a daily basis and hence we have to use our time off wisely to move our bodies as much as we can. The benefit of linking exercise to family- or friend-based activities is that you get to spend quality time together as well as burn calories.

If you find that your kids are already active over the weekend but you struggle to fit in some physical activity, the best thing you can do is to add a regular walk either on Sunday morning or Sunday afternoon. Similar to the way in which we schedule all our other 'to do's' each day, a walk or gym session every Sunday needs to ultimately become a core part of our Sundays if we are to reach our exercise targets in the midst of frantic weekdays.

Sunday exercise ideas

1. Schedule in a regular long walk (3–4 hours) with friends and family and enjoy lunch on the way.

2. Join a bushwalking club, the local surf club or other club and take advantage of the active recreational options they offer.

3. Meet friends for a walk, lunch or brunch.

4. Begin your Sundays with a long bike ride or run as you prepare for the day's events.

5. In the warmer weather meet friends for a swim, surf or sail if you are based near the coast.

❊ *Think outside the square when it comes to your Sunday activities. Try an all-day walk, spend the day at the beach, climb a mountain or head to a national park for a picnic. No matter where you go, you will be more active than if you had stayed at home.*

❖ *Stay well clear of shopping centres during the busiest weekend times. The noise, encouragement to spend and over consume and the throng of busy people rushing around is enough to leave you stressed and frazzled on what should be the calmest day of the week.*

Implement a technology ban

It does not matter whether it is the phone, television, internet or social media – all forms of electronic entertainment act to prevent genuine communication between individuals. Even if you only switch off for a few hours each week, make a commitment to switch off on Sunday and notice how much better you feel when you return to work on Monday – you will feel as if you have actually had a break.

Perhaps the most important time to consider doing this is on Sunday night. While Sunday evening is prime-time viewing for a number of television shows, it is also the time in which you can get many things organised for the week ahead. If you still decide to spend an hour or two watching television on Sunday night, use the time in the ad breaks to get organised for Monday to make sure that you head off to bed at a decent hour so you can start the week feeling energised and refreshed.

❖ *Always aim to withdraw from social media and technology at least an hour before you go to bed at night to help your brain relax and wind down to sleep.*

Go light with your calories on Sunday night

Of course it is the weekend, and there are likely to have been a number of eating occasions in which you have eaten more than you usually would. But rather than wait until another Monday morning to start your diet, you need to get back on track Sunday night. No more blocks of chocolate or heavy desserts just because you have the Sunday night blues; if you are serious about taking control of your weight, you need to go light on Sunday night.

This may mean soup, salad or a light grill, but sticking to a meal of less than 300 calories will ensure that you start your Monday feeling light, fantastic and ready to keep the focus on your diet and exercise regime for at least the first half of the week.

Light Sunday night dinner suggestions

100g grilled white fish with vegetables

Bowl of vegetable soup

1-egg omelette

Warm chicken salad

Frittata and salad

❖ *One of the biggest issues when it comes to weight control is not getting enough sleep. Make it a priority to have an early night on Sunday so you can start the new week refreshed and well rested.*

SUNDAY VEGETABLE TIP:

Always add a vegetable-based soup or salad to your Sunday night meal to help keep your calorie intake low after the weekend's treats.

Sunday meal plans

Breakfast
Banana Nut Pancakes (page 81) OR small serve of pancakes with small skim coffee

Lunch
Chicken caesar salad with 100g grilled chicken breast, 1 slice 97% fat-free bacon, 2 tbsp low-fat caesar dressing and lettuce OR Grilled Salmon with Coleslaw (page 82)

Dinner
Creamy Broccoli and Cauliflower Soup (page 84)

Breakfast
Healthy Benedict (page 81) OR 1 slice toast with 2 eggs and 1 piece lean bacon with mushrooms and tomato

Lunch
Toasted sandwich with 50g 97% fat-free ham and 1 slice light Jarlsberg cheese on grain bread, 1 small banana OR Baked Chicken with Spinach Salad (page 83)

Dinner
Salmon and Ricotta Tart (page 85) with 2 cups salad OR 100g grilled salmon with 2 cups roasted vegetables

Breakfast
2 poached eggs on 1 slice grain bread with 1 small glass (200ml) orange juice or small skim coffee

Lunch

Light Chicken Pie (page 83) with 2 cups salad or vegetables

Dinner

Sweet Potato Soup (page 86)

Breakfast

Egg Fry-Up (page 82) OR Parmesan Eggs (below) with small skim milk coffee

Lunch

Mexican Steak Wraps (page 84) OR steak sandwich OR plain hamburger with salad

Dinner

2 Salmon Patties (page 86) with 2 cups salad or vegetables OR 150g grilled white fish with salad or vegetables

SUNDAY BREAKFAST

PARMESAN EGGS

4 roma tomatoes, chopped

1 tbsp olive oil

8 eggs

¾ cup low-fat milk

½ cup Parmesan cheese

½ cup light sour cream

4 slices sourdough bread

1 Roast tomatoes with a drizzle of olive oil for 20 minutes at 180°C.

2 Whisk eggs with milk. Add Parmesan and sour cream and cook in a frying pan over medium heat with a little olive oil.

3 Toast bread and serve with eggs and tomatoes.

Serves 4

BANANA NUT PANCAKES

1 cup cooked quinoa

4 egg whites

½ cup low-fat milk

2 tsp brown sugar

½ tsp vanilla extract

1 banana, sliced

canola oil spray

½ cup Greek-style yoghurt

½ cup chopped walnuts

1 tsp maple syrup

1 Whisk quinoa with egg whites, milk, sugar, vanilla extract and ¼ banana.

2 Spray frying pan with canola oil and divide batter into 2 pancakes. Cook each pancake over medium heat for 3 minutes on each side.

3 Serve with extra banana, yoghurt, a sprinkle of walnuts and a drizzle of maple syrup.

Serves 2

HEALTHY BENEDICT

2 tbsp light sour cream

2 tsp reduced-fat milk

1 tsp Dijon mustard

1 tsp olive oil

1 cup button mushrooms, sliced

2 tbsp chopped shallots

2 cups baby spinach leaves

4 eggs

2 large slices sourdough bread, toasted

1 In a bowl combine sour cream, milk and mustard. Set aside.

2 Heat oil in a frying pan over medium heat. Add mushrooms and shallots and cook until mushrooms are golden brown. Add spinach and cook until spinach starts to wilt.

3 Half-fill a saucepan with water and bring to the boil and then reduce to a simmer. Crack each egg into a bowl separately and then slide one by one into water and cook until yolks begin to thicken.

4 Toast bread and top with ½ mushroom mix, 2 eggs and drizzle with sauce.

Serves 2

EGG FRY-UP

1 large potato, cut into small cubes

olive oil

2 spring onions, finely chopped

2 cups chopped English spinach

40g shaved Parmesan cheese

4 eggs

2 tbsp sweet chilli sauce

1 Cook potato in 1 tbsp oil in a frying pan over medium heat.

2 Combine 1 tsp olive oil with spring onion. Add spinach and Parmesan and lightly cook with potatoes.

3 Half-fill a saucepan with water and bring to the boil and then reduce to a simmer. Crack each egg into a bowl separately and then slide one by one into water and cook until yolks begin to thicken.

4 Serve spinach and potato salad topped with poached egg. Serve with sweet chilli sauce as desired.

Serves 4

SUNDAY LUNCHES

GRILLED SALMON WITH COLESLAW

4 x 150g salmon fillets

½ cabbage, shredded

½ red cabbage, shredded

2 medium carrots, grated

2 sticks celery, grated

½ cup egg mayonnaise

½ lemon

1 Grill salmon steaks under medium heat.

2 Combine salad ingredients. Mix through mayonnaise and add lemon juice.

3 Serve salmon on coleslaw bed.

Serves 4

BAKED CHICKEN WITH SPINACH SALAD

1kg chicken breast fillets

2 cups buttermilk

2 tbsp honey

2 garlic cloves, finely chopped

1½ cups multigrain breadcrumbs

4 cups baby spinach leaves

1 bunch cooked asparagus, cut into 3cm lengths

1 punnet cherry tomatoes

1 tbsp olive oil

balsamic vinegar

1 Slice chicken into strips and place in large bowl.

2 Whisk buttermilk, honey and garlic together and pour over chicken. Leave to marinate for at least 2 hours.

3 Preheat oven to 200°C. Remove chicken from marinade, coat with breadcrumbs and bake for 30–40 minutes.

4 While chicken is cooking, combine spinach leaves, asparagus and tomatoes and dress with mix of olive oil and balsamic vinegar.

Serves 4

LIGHT CHICKEN PIE

500g chicken breast fillets

1 medium onion, finely chopped

2 carrots, chopped

olive oil

¼ cup flour

2½ cups reduced-fat milk

1 cup frozen peas

6–8 sheets filo pastry

1 Pan-fry or grill chicken. Set aside.

2 Cook onion and carrot in 1 tbsp olive oil in a saucepan over medium heat. Add flour, stir for 1 minute, then gradually stir in milk. Cook until mixture thickens. Remove from heat.

3 Add peas and chicken and pour into a pie dish.

4 Preheat oven to 180°C. Brush pastry sheets with a little olive oil, layer over pie dish and trim off excess. Bake for 20–25 minutes, until golden.

Serves 4–6

MEXICAN STEAK WRAPS

750g lean rump steak, sliced

1 cup taco sauce

1 brown onion, sliced

2 zucchinis, sliced

1 tsp olive oil

1 red capsicum, sliced

6–8 mushrooms, sliced

½ cup brown sugar

4 small flour or corn tortillas, warmed

2 tbsps reduced-fat sour cream

1 Combine steak and taco sauce in a bowl and marinate for 5–10 minutes.

2 Stir fry onion and zucchini in olive oil until brown. Add capsicum, mushrooms, sugar and ½ cup water. Stir fry until sugar has caramelised. Set aside.

3 Stir fry steak strips until cooked through. Combine with vegetables.

4 To serve, place vegetable and steak mixture into tortillas. Add sour cream.

Serves 4

SUNDAY DINNERS

CREAMY BROCCOLI AND CAULIFLOWER SOUP

2 tsp olive oil

1 large onion, chopped

1 clove garlic, crushed

500g broccoli florets

500g cauliflower florets

2 cups salt-reduced vegetable stock

2 cups water

1½ cups low-fat milk

1 Heat olive oil in a large saucepan. Add onion and garlic and sauté until soft.

2 Add broccoli, cauliflower, stock and 2 cups water. Bring to boil, reduce heat, cover and simmer for 15 minutes.

3 Remove from heat and allow to cool slightly, then purée until smooth.

4 Add milk and blend until combined.

5 Return to saucepan and reheat before serving.

Serves 4

SALMON AND RICOTTA TART

cooking oil spray

4 sheets filo pastry

200g smoked salmon, roughly chopped

150g low-fat ricotta cheese

3 tbsp dill, finely chopped

2 eggs, lightly beaten

½ cup low-fat milk

4 cups salad leaves

1 Preheat oven to 180°C. Coat a 20cm baking tin with cooking oil spray. Line the base with 1 sheet of pastry and lightly coat with spray before placing the next sheet of pastry on top. Continue with remaining pastry sheets. Place tin on a baking tray and bake for 8 minutes, until lightly golden.

2 Combine the remaining ingredients in a bowl, seasoning well with salt and pepper. Gently pour the salmon mixture into the cooked pastry case.

3 Reduce oven temperature to 160°C and bake for 35 minutes, or until the salmon filling is set. Serve with salad.

Serves 4

SALMON PATTIES

500g sweet potato

415g can no added salt red salmon, drained

2 egg whites, lightly beaten

4 spring onions, sliced

1 red capsicum, finely chopped

2 cups multigrain breadcrumbs

2 tbsp chopped fresh dill

1–2 tbsp lemon juice

olive oil spray

1 Cook sweet potato in oven at 180°C for 30–40 minutes until soft then mash until smooth.

2 Combine sweet potato, salmon, egg whites, spring onion, capsicum, breadcrumbs, dill and lemon juice in a bowl.

3 Divide mixture into 8 portions and shape into flat patties. Put on a baking tray lined with non-stick baking paper and refrigerate for 30 minutes, until firm. Preheat oven to 220°C.

4 Lightly spray a non-stick frying pan with olive oil and warm over medium heat until hot. Fry the patties in batches until golden brown on both sides, transfer to the oven and cook for 10–15 minutes, until heated through. Serve patties with side salad.

Serves 4

SWEET POTATO SOUP

1 onion, sliced

2 gloves garlic

1 tbsp olive oil

500g sweet potato, cut into cubes

3½ cups salt-reduced vegetable stock

1 large zucchini

1 Brown the onion and garlic in olive oil in a saucepan over medium heat.

2 Add sweet potato and vegetable stock and cook for 20–25 minutes.

3 Grate zucchini into soup just before serving.

Serves 4–6

RESET MONDAY

The Monday plan

1. Start the day right.

2. Get up early.

3. Start the day with some exercise

4. Take time out to plan and make your lists.

5. Have a low-calorie day.

❖ *Enjoy your breakfast rather than scoffing it. Savour your morning brew and listen to some upbeat, inspirational music with the aim of easing into and enjoying your Monday.*

Start the day right

If your Monday morning routinely begins with you rushing out the door with nothing but your laptop and a cup of instant coffee, the chance is slim that you will be feeling good about your week and ready to eat well. If, however, you take time to ease into your day, enjoy a light, 'detox'-style breakfast and cup of herbal tea, you will start your Monday in the right mindset to eat well and control your weight. This is likely to mean that you will need to get out of bed a little earlier to ensure you have time for breakfast, and plan beforehand what foods you need to grab to eat well during the day.

Think about the way you begin your day and work towards developing some rituals that will help get you into the right mindset for a healthy, organised week. Daily rituals not only help to structure our lives, but they also help bring small amounts of pleasure into our world on a daily basis.

Powerful morning rituals include starting the day with a few yoga poses or stretching followed by a cup of herbal tea and a nourishing breakfast. Starting the day – especially Monday – with these rituals at the forefront of your mind will further support your commitment to health and wellbeing for the remainder of the day, and ideally the rest of the week once these morning health rituals become long-term health habits.

Sample daily rituals

Get up and stretch for 5 minutes.

Enjoy a cup of herbal tea while making your weekly 'to do' list.

Eat a protein-rich breakfast while catching up on the overnight news.

Take a brisk walk with the family pet.

Read from a motivational book or listen to your favourite song on the way to work.

❀ *Hot water with lemon, ginger and a little honey makes a wonderful brew to start your day with and represents a powerful hydration ritual.*

The other crucial morning ritual is to ensure that you consume a nourishing breakfast as early as possible. Waiting until you get to the office at 9am is leaving it too late – the earlier you eat your breakfast, the better it is for your metabolism. Your Monday breakfast and your Monday meals in general should be light, and based around plenty of low-calorie fresh fruit and vegetables to help keep your calorie intake low and reset your metabolism after the sins of the weekend. Light Monday breakfast options include a meal replacement shake, some natural yoghurt and fruit or a light egg scramble.

Get up early

❋ *The early bird simply gets more done.*

Successful people know that getting up early means they have more time in their day to complete the things they need to do to continually move forward in life. They understand that all of us are generally playing a time game, with time being one of our most precious resources. If you consider that getting out of bed an hour earlier on weekdays will give you an extra two whole days each year, imagine how much more you could achieve if you got up even earlier.

Whether an early start helps to get extra chores completed, allows time for you to exercise or simply represents an hour or two when you can enjoy some peace and quiet, the feeling of starting your day gently, without rushing, is a sure-fire way to start your week in the right frame of mind for a successful, fulfilling week.

Getting up early on Monday means you have time to start the day with ease and grace – to eat breakfast and fit in some exercise. Often we focus on the fact that we are either a 'morning person' or we are not, but the truth is that we can program ourselves to be a morning person, especially when we can see the benefits of doing so.

❧ *It takes 3 months for a new routine to become a habit, so keep setting that alarm 30 or 60 minutes earlier for Monday morning so you can program yourself to become a morning person.*

Start the day with some exercise

❧ *Make it a habit to begin each Monday with a brisk walk or light jog. Weekly habits form the basis of long-term lifestyle success.*

For many people looking to start the week right, this means beginning with some exercise. In fact, there is no better way to begin a Monday than with a brisk walk or run to kick-start your metabolism and get you in the right frame of mind for eating well and maintaining your exercise program.

One of the biggest issues when it comes to committing to a concerted effort to factor regular exercise into your lifestyle is the belief pattern associated with regular training. Exercise does not necessarily mean numerous uncomfortable, sweaty hours spent at the gym – it can simply mean walking to work or getting off the bus or train one stop earlier. Making a commitment to taking small but regular exercise on a daily basis is often the difference between controlling your weight or not.

On Monday mornings your ideal exercise scenario may mean a session with a trainer to start the week on the right foot, or a quick walk before breakfast. Alternatively, it may mean making the commitment to walk to work, or at least getting off the bus or train a stop earlier so that you are forced to move more than you usually would. Whatever your ideal scenario exercise is, it needs to be scheduled into your Monday morning.

Take time out to plan and make your lists

❧ *One of the most powerful predictors of whether someone will achieve their goals is whether they have been written down or not.*

Another powerful Monday habit that will serve you well over many years is to start each week with a clear, written 'to do' list. Operating in the same way as goals do to help direct and guide behaviour, writing a 'to do' list helps keep you on track with the bigger picture plans you have for yourself. A list helps to focus your behaviour and choices, especially during times in which it is easy to get distracted; it also helps you get to the end of the week feeling as though you have achieved something you set out to do. So, get into the habit of sitting for 5 minutes each Monday morning and making a note of the key things you want to have achieved by the end of the week. You will be surprised how much easier it is to stay focused when you know what you are supposed to be concentrating on.

Once you have your list completed each week, place it where you will view it regularly, whether it be at your desk, in the bathroom or as a reminder on your mobile phone. Try to take time each day to consider the progress you have made with your 'to do' list – you will be surprised how much more you have achieved each week once you actually write down what your goals are and monitor your progress.

Have a low-calorie day

❧ *Aiming for one low-calorie day each week is a great way to remind you of how little food we really need. As a rule of thumb, make sure that all your meals on a Monday are based around fresh fruits and vegetables to keep your calorie intake low.*

Chances are that, come Monday morning, you are already well aware of the sins of the weekend and this means that you need a day of light eating to get back on track. Think an entire day of light salads, soups, juices and low-carbohydrate food options to not only cut back on calories but to fill your body with nutritious light food options. Plenty of fresh fruits and vegetables will not only help to clean out your digestive tract and drop any extra fluid weight you may have gained over the weekend, but it will remind you of how much better you feel when you only eat unprocessed natural foods.

A light day of eating means cutting back on the carbohydrate-rich foods, including bread, rice, cereal and pasta. While there can be concern expressed with diet plans that aggressively cut carbohydrate-based foods out of the diet, when carbohydrates are reduced for short periods of time there are no associated health risks. A day of lighter eating simply means that fewer calories are consumed and the carbohydrates are consumed via fresh fruits, vegetables and some light dairy foods.

A day of light eating – without the sugar, caffeine and processed carbohydrates – also plays a powerful role in reminding us how reliant we tend to become on these non-nutritious foods and stimulants for energy. Once we have a day without them we allow the body's natural physiology to return to baseline and find that our appetite is better managed, we sleep better and are far less vulnerable to the energy highs and lows that tend to accompany frequent consumption of these foods and drinks.

Monday snack list

A piece of fruit

30g mixed nuts

2 tbsp hummus with cut-up vegetables

20g roasted chickpeas

2 cups of natural popcorn

❀ *If you do feel hungry between your meals, on a Monday grab an extra piece of fruit or a small handful of nuts to keep your hunger at bay until your next meal.*

MONDAY VEGETABLE TIP:
Start each Monday with a container of chopped-up salad vegetables that you can keep on your desk at work to munch on throughout the day.

❀ *Love your coffee? While a coffee a day will not hurt you, every so often try cutting the coffee out for a day and instead enjoy herbal tea. Taking a break from caffeine occasionally is a good way to ensure we do not become too reliant on it.*

Monday exercise ideas

1. Schedule a training session for first thing Monday morning.

2. Walk or run at lunchtime.

3. Add in a 20–30 minute high-intensity interval session at the gym.

4. Walk home from work.

5. Join an exercise class after work or midmorning after the school drop-off.

❀ *Always know what you will be eating for the following day's lunch. A great option is to use Monday night's leftovers as a base for your lunch on Tuesday.*

Monday meal plans

Breakfast
Protein Smoothie (page 96) OR meal replacement shake or bar

Lunch
Vegetable Salad with Cottage Cheese (page 97) OR 100g pink or red salmon (or turkey or chicken) with large mixed green salad with ¼ avocado

Dinner
Baked Fish (page 99) with 2 cups vegetables OR 150g grilled white fish with dry roasted eggplant, zucchini, pumpkin and red capsicum and 1 tbsp low-fat hummus

Breakfast
High-protein Cereal Mix (page 96) OR ¾ cup bran cereal or 1 multigrain Weetbix with 1 cup low-fat milk and 1 nectarine or peach

Lunch
Antioxidant Salad (page 98) OR 2 California sushi rolls with a bowl of miso soup and small apple or orange

Dinner
Hearty Dinner Soup (page 100) OR 2 cups vegetable soup

Breakfast
Monday Reset Juice (page 97) OR 250ml low-fat milk and ½ cup berry smoothie

Lunch
2 leftover Salmon Patties from Sunday night (page 86) with 2 cups mixed salad OR Quinoa and Feta Salad (page 98)

Dinner
Spinach Pie (page 99) with 2 cups salad OR 2-egg vegetable omelette

Breakfast
Breakfast Mess (page 96) OR egg-white omelette with 1–2 cups mixed vegetables

Lunch
Spinach Pie (page 99) with 2 cups salad OR 95g can tuna with 130g can corn and 2 cups mixed salad with ¼ avocado

Dinner
Prawns with Roasted Vegetables (page 100) OR 10–12 grilled prawns with 2 cups vegetables roasted with 1 tbsp olive oil

PROTEIN SMOOTHIE

1 cup blueberries

½ cup ice

½ cup Greek-style yoghurt

1 tbsp vanilla protein powder

⅓ cup low-fat milk

Blend all ingredients together for a delicious breakfast smoothie.

Serves 1

HIGH-PROTEIN CEREAL MIX

½ cup cooked rolled oats or bran cereal

½ cup mixed berries

½ cup low-fat cottage cheese

Sprinkle of cinnamon

Mix cereal, berries and cottage cheese together. Sprinkle with cinnamon.

Serves 1

BREAKFAST MESS

3 egg whites

1 egg yolk

½ cup low-fat milk

cooking oil spray

1 cup mixed vegetables

¼ cup cottage or soft goat's cheese

1 tbsp sweet chilli sauce

1   Whisk eggs with milk. Place frying pan over medium heat, spray with oil and lightly cook vegetables for 2–3 minutes.

2   Pour egg mix over vegetables and cook until set. Sprinkle with cheese and serve with sweet chilli sauce.

Serves 1

MONDAY RESET JUICE

3 oranges

3 sticks celery

1 large carrot

1 beetroot (head)

small handful of mint leaves

Juice all ingredients together for a Monday detox juice.

Serves 2

MONDAY LUNCHES

VEGETABLE SALAD WITH COTTAGE CHEESE

1 tbsp olive oil

1 tbsp white wine vinegar

1 tbsp lemon juice

4 asparagus spears, trimmed

1 carrot, sliced

1 small zucchini, sliced into ribbons

1 small red capsicum, sliced

10 snow peas

½ cup cooked cannellini beans

3 tbsp cottage or soft goat's cheese

1 Mix together oil, vinegar and lemon juice.

2 Mix vegetables in a bowl, pour over dressing and serve with cheese.

Serves 1

ANTIOXIDANT SALAD

50g Danish feta cheese, crumbled

1 nashi pear, sliced

mixed lettuce leaves

4 roma tomatoes, quartered

1 red onion, chopped

2 handfuls dried cranberries

1 red capsicum, sliced

1 Lebanese cucumber

Toss all ingredients together for an antioxidant-rich salad.

Serves 2

QUINOA AND FETA SALAD

1 cup green beans, lightly steamed

1 Lebanese cucumber, cut into rounds

½ cup Danish feta cheese, crumbled

⅓ cup pistachio nuts or walnuts

¼ cup sultanas

1 cup cooked quinoa

1 tbsp olive oil

pinch of salt

Mix salad ingredients with quinoa. Dress with olive oil and season with salt.

Serves 2

BAKED FISH

2 tsp honey

1 tsp peanut oil

1 small hot chilli, finely sliced

1 tsp grated ginger

1 tsp lemon juice

1 tbsp salt-reduced soy sauce

1 kg firm white fish fillets

1 Preheat oven to 200°C.

2 Place honey, peanut oil, chilli, ginger, lemon juice and soy sauce in a screw-top jar and shake well.

3 Brush fish with dressing and bake for 20 minutes on a greased oven tray.

4 Serve with fresh salad.

Serves 4

SPINACH PIE

6–8 cups or 2 x 150g bags of baby spinach leaves

2 eggs

250g low-fat ricotta cheese

200g reduced-fat feta cheese

2 spring onions, chopped

olive oil spray

4 sheets filo pastry

1 Preheat oven to 180°C.

2 Lightly wilt spinach leaves in water in microwave. Chop roughly.

3 Mix eggs, ricotta, feta and chopped onion in a bowl. Fold in spinach.

4 Spray baking tray with oil and fill with cheese mixture.

5 Top with filo and bake for 30 minutes, until pastry is browned.

6 Serve with large green salad.

Serves 4

PRAWNS WITH ROASTED VEGETABLES

1 beetroot

2 red onions, sliced

1kg jap pumpkin, diced

1 eggplant, diced

2 zucchinis, sliced into diagonal chunks

2 tbsp olive oil

15–20 cooked king prawns

2 tsp balsamic vinegar

1 Preheat oven to 180°C. Wrap beetroot in foil and bake for 45 minutes.

2 Place remaining vegetables in baking dish, drizzle with oil and bake for 30 minutes, or until tender.

3 Mix cooked vegetables together and serve with fresh prawns and drizzle of balsamic vinegar.

Serves 2–4

HEARTY DINNER SOUP

2 tsp olive oil

1 onion, finely chopped

1 leek, thinly sliced

2 cups salt-reduced vegetable stock

2 x 400g cans diced tomatoes

1 carrot, peeled and cut into 1cm cubes

500g pumpkin, cut into 1 cm cubes

250g sweet potato, cut into cubes

½ stick celery, chopped

1 broccoli head, steamed

1 Heat olive oil and onion in a large saucepan over low heat. Add leek and gently cook until soft. Add stock, 3 cups water, tomatoes, carrot, pumpkin, sweet potato and celery.

2 Bring to the boil, reduce heat and simmer for 10 minutes.

3 Top with steamed broccoli and serve.

Serves 6–8

TRAINING TUESDAY

The Tuesday plan

1. Start with a protein-rich breakfast.

2. One milk coffee a day.

3. Take charge of lunch.

4. Training: 'Go hard or go home.'

5. Always start Tuesday with a workout.

❀ *Tuesdays are perhaps the most crucial day of the week when it comes to weight loss.*

Start with a protein-rich breakfast

While breakfast cereal, toast and fruit are all healthy breakfast choices, their high carbohydrate content relative to the amount of protein they contain does not necessarily make them the best choice for weight control. Instead, choosing protein-rich breakfast options such as eggs, cottage cheese, a protein or meal replacement shake or even lean meat or fish, and basing your breakfast around these foods, is more likely to give you the 15–20g of total protein you need to help maintain sugar levels and your appetite throughout the morning.

The best 300-calorie (20g) protein breakfasts

1 slice grain toast + 2 eggs

1 slice grain toast + 130g can baked beans + 1 slice cheese

3–4 corn crackers + ½ cup cottage cheese + tomato

Wholegrain wrap + 1 egg + 1 slice lean bacon

2 slices grain bread + 50g ham + 20g cheese

½ cup bran cereal + 1 cup high-protein yoghurt (>10g protein/serve)

⅓ cup oats + 1 cup low-fat milk + 1 tsp protein powder

20g protein powder + 200ml milk + ½ banana

150g thick yoghurt + 20g protein + ½ cup berries

1 slice grain toast + 50g smoked salmon + ¼ avocado

❖ *Ensuring that your breakfast contains 20g of protein is a great way to help control your insulin levels and manage your hunger throughout the day.*

One milk coffee a day

There is nothing wrong with enjoying a cup of coffee, but a more common scenario is that busy workers drink milk-based coffee such as cappuccinos, lattes and flat whites nonstop throughout the day. The issue with this is that constantly sipping on milk-based coffee results in a constant release of insulin, elevated levels of which act to prevent fat being burnt in the body. A second issue with drinking large volumes of coffee throughout the day is that we tend not to feel hungry when we naturally would. In turn, this means that we do not eat regular meals and snacks throughout the day and are then more likely to overeat at night.

If you love your coffee, come Tuesday, limit yourself to one milk-based coffee each day. If you enjoy your coffee black, then drinking 2–4 cups of coffee throughout the day will ensure that your caffeine intake is kept moderately controlled. The next rule is to only order a small coffee. And finally, pay attention to the times when you choose to drink your coffee. Starting the day with a cappuccino followed by another just an hour or so later means that you have not left enough time in between to let your digestive hormones return to normal. So always make sure you leave at least 2–3 hours between each coffee. If you must drink something in between, try herbal tea or water, which do not contain any calories.

✤ *The average small coffee contains as many calories as a slice of bread, so make sure you include this in your daily calorie intake.*

A piccolo contains less than half as many calories as a regular coffee and is a great option for coffee lovers.

Take charge of lunch

Too often in the working week lunch is simply not given enough attention. It is regularly skipped and replaced with coffee and snacks later in the day, eaten haphazardly in front of a computer or picked up on the run, and it ends up being a high-fat, high-calorie choice that leaves us feeling full, sludgy and heavy all afternoon. It may surprise you to learn that it is actually our lunch choices that tend to predict our dietary success through the working week. If we get our lunch choice right, we are far less likely to snack on non-nutritious, high-calorie foods throughout the day, which also means that we are less likely to arrive home from work absolutely starving and overeat then.

Getting the right nutritional balance at work is not easy. You do have to get organised and know exactly what mix of foods to work towards to get your balance right, but once you have this knowledge you will use this skill forever.

The classic, 'healthy' lunchtime staples of sandwiches, salads and sushi, while seemingly all good choices, fail to tick all the key nutritional boxes we need at this time of day to help us feel full and satisfied. Plain salads lack the calories to keep us satisfied throughout the afternoon, while sushi lacks the protein and bulk to keep us going for more than an hour or two.

When it comes to making the best lunch choices, the easiest thing to do is to break it down into key sections:

1. Low GI carbohydrates for energy.

2. Lean protein for fullness.

3. 2–3 cups of vegetables or salad for nutrition and appetite control.

To make sure that you do not run the risk of late afternoon hunger and sugar cravings, check that your lunch contains each of these core components.

❖ *Get into the habit of chopping extra salad vegetables into a container each evening and taking them with you to snack on throughout the day at work.*

❀ *Sandwiches are often too large to eat in one sitting. Instead, split them in half and have an early lunch, and save the other half for later in the afternoon as a filling snack to keep you going until dinnertime.*

Top Tuesday lunches

1 California sushi roll with miso soup and edamame beans

½ large salad and meat wrap or sandwich

½ cup cooked brown rice with meat/chicken and vegetable stir fry

Lamb, sweet potato and rocket salad

½ cup pasta with tuna and salad

❀ *Never be afraid to make special lunch requests when you are spending your lunchtimes in meetings. The better you eat, the better you will perform.*

❀ *Ever thought of starting a 'lunch club' at work so you can take turns at preparing a healthy lunch each week for your colleagues? Then on the fifth day, you can enjoy a lunch out together.*

❀ *Do you exercise in the afternoon and need a filling snack to help you make it through until dinner? These are your best options.*

Tuesday snack list

Nut-based snack bar

Protein shake with skim milk

150g natural yoghurt with ½ cup berries

4 rye crackers with ½ cup cottage cheese

1 piece of fruit with 20g cheese

Training: 'Go hard or go home'

In an ideal world we would make it to the gym each evening after work, spend a good hour there before returning home to a dinner of chicken breast and vegetables. Unfortunately, with the demands of a busy life, many of us are lucky to make it to the gym once or twice a week and dinner is likely to be an Asian takeaway picked up on the way home. For this reason, when we do find ourselves with time to get to the gym, or aggressively schedule our training sessions into our schedules so we can get there, we have to go hard. A 30-minute walk or class does not cut it – when we train, we have to make it a priority to burn serious calories and make a real dent in our metabolic rate. This means pushing ourselves to the limit, doing a longer session than we usually would, doing extra cardio on top of our class, or going for a run both in the morning and at night. Tuesday is the perfect day to do this.

Always start Tuesday with a workout

While Monday may seem like the best time to begin your training for the week, too many of us skip this session after a big weekend. If you make it to the gym or go for a run on a Monday, well done, but if you know you are often too tired and miss out on training sessions on Mondays, schedule your workouts for Tuesday.

The best time to train is always the time when you are most likely to do it, but for most of us it is best to train first thing in the morning to ensure that the demands of the day do not take over. Start your commitment to Training Tuesday by always beginning your day with a 20 or 30 minute walk, run or gym session. If you can afford it, book a trainer or schedule a session with friends. The more committed you are, the less likely it is that you will cancel or not turn up.

Keep in mind that training does not necessarily have to mean a trip to the gym. It could simply mean that you walk to work or get off the bus or train a few stops earlier. Indeed, this is often a far more viable option for city workers and a simple way to incorporate your activity into your day without even noticing it.

❖ *Need to walk more? Spend time putting your favourite music or podcast on your iPod so you always have something entertaining to listen to.*

Tuesday exercise ideas

1. Look for a local boxing class or an outdoor group training program.

2. Sign up to a 6–8 week intensive training program.

3. Sign up for a fun run or local triathlon and set a training plan to complement that.

4. Start a Tuesday run or walking club at work.

5. Include 2 short but intense training sessions in your Tuesday schedule.

TUESDAY VEGETABLE TIP:

Keep some tomatoes, capsicums and cucumbers at work to add to your lunch sandwich or salad to bulk up your meal without the extra calories.

❊ *If you are spending the night in on a Tuesday, allocate an hour or two to prepare a couple of healthy meals for lunch and/or dinner for the week ahead.*

Tuesday meal plans

Breakfast
Breakfast Sandwich (page 110) OR 1 slice wholegrain bread with 130g (½ cup) baked beans and 1 slice reduced-fat cheese

Lunch
1 wholegrain wrap with 100g sliced turkey breast with rocket and 1 piece of fruit OR Qunioa and Prawn Salad (page 112)

Dinner
Sesame Chicken (page 114) OR 100g chicken breast with 1 tsp sweet chilli sauce with 100g roasted sweet potato and green beans

Breakfast

Breakfast Omelette (page 110) OR 2 poached eggs on 1 slice wholegrain bread and 1 × 200ml glass vegetable or tomato juice

Lunch

Sesame Chicken (page 114) OR ¾ cup brown rice mixed with 100g chicken breast, red capsicum, snow peas, broccoli and 2 tbsp sweet chilli sauce

Dinner

5-Minute Dinner Pasta (page 114) with 2 cups salad OR ½ cup quinoa with 100g salmon and 2 cups vegetables

Breakfast

Breakfast Energy Shake (page 111) OR skim milk smoothie with banana and 20g protein powder

Lunch

Leftover 5-Minute Dinner Pasta (page 114) OR ¾ cup cooked pasta with 95g small can tuna, 4 olives, 1 chopped tomato, 1 tsp olive oil OR Salmon and Pumpkin Salad (page 113)

Dinner

Curried Fish (page 115) OR 150g grilled white fish with 1 small jacket potato and roasted pumpkin and zucchini OR Chicken and Bean Soup (page 113)

Breakfast

Breakfast Soup (page 111) OR wholegrain wrap with 1 egg, sliced tomato, rocket, 1 slice 97% fat-free bacon and 1 tbsp low-fat mayonnaise

Lunch

Chicken Salad (page 112) OR turkey or chicken and salad wrap

Dinner

Satay Roo (page 115) with roasted vegetables OR 100g grilled steak or lamb with 2 cups vegetables roasted with 1 tbsp olive oil

TUESDAY BREAKFASTS

BREAKFAST OMELETTE

3 egg whites

1 egg yolk

1 tsp olive oil

1 cup baby spinach leaves

3 cherry tomatoes, chopped

¼ cup cottage cheese

20g feta or reduced-fat cheddar cheese

1 slice grain or sourdough bread

1 Whisk eggs together and set aside.

2 Over medium heat, heat oil and add spinach and cook until tender. Add eggs and flip into an omelette. Once cooked, add tomatoes and cottage cheese.

3 Serve on toasted bread.

Serves 1

BREAKFAST SANDWICH

2 slices grain bread or small wholegrain wrap

1 tsp extra-light cream cheese

100g lean turkey, ham, smoked salmon or sardines

½ tomato, sliced

1 slice light Jarlsberg cheese

Spread bread with cream cheese. Stack ingredients and serve toasted if desired.

Serves 1

BREAKFAST ENERGY SHAKE

1 egg

200ml low-fat milk

1 scoop vanilla whey protein powder

1 tsp honey

1 banana

¼ cup frozen berries

1 heaped tbsp low-fat vanilla yoghurt

Whiz all ingredients in blender until smooth for a perfect balance of carbs and protein for breakfast.

Serves 1

BREAKFAST SOUP

1L water

400g chicken breast fillet

⅔ cup brown rice

3 diced shallots

4 sticks celery

2 cups green beans

2 cups shredded lettuce

Place all ingredients in saucepan and simmer over low heat for 40 minutes. Season with salt and pepper. The soup will keep for 3–4 days and makes a great protein-rich, gluten-free breakfast or lunch.

Serves 4–6

QUINOA AND PRAWN SALAD

32 green prawns

1 tbsp sesame or peanut oil

1 cup quinoa

1 red capsicum, seeded and diced

2 sticks celery, finely chopped

2 spring onions, finely chopped

1 punnet cherry tomatoes, chopped

2 tbsp sweet chilli sauce

1 Sear prawns in a little oil over medium heat until they turn pink, then remove from frying pan.

2 Combine quinoa with 2 cups water in saucepan or shallow frying pan, bring to the boil and cook until water is absorbed and quinoa is clear.

3 Stir in remaining ingredients, including cooked prawns, and serve.

Serves 4

CHICKEN SALAD

500g chicken breast fillets

1 tbsp olive oil

1 tbsp Dijon mustard

2 cups sugar snap peas

8 cups mixed lettuce leaves

8 radishes, sliced

2 carrots, grated

1 red capsicum, finely sliced

1 Grill chicken and cut into slices.

2 Mix olive oil and mustard together.

3 Lightly steam peas.

4 Mix all salad ingredients and top with Dijon mustard dressing.

Serves 4

SALMON AND PUMPKIN SALAD

100g fresh or canned salmon

1 cup steamed or roasted pumpkin cubes

½ cup fresh or canned corn

2 cups mixed lettuce leaves

½ Lebanese cucumber, sliced

150g or 1 cup baby roma or cherry tomatoes

2 tsp red wine vinegar

Mix salad ingredients together and dress with small amount of vinegar.

Serves 1

CHICKEN AND BEAN SOUP

1 tbsp olive oil

½ red onion, diced

1kg chicken breast fillet, cubed

2 cups salt-reduced chicken stock

250g packet frozen chopped spinach

1 can red kidney beans

1 can cannellini beans

1 can white beans

1 cup water

1 Heat olive oil and onion over medium heat in a large soup pot. Add chicken, stir to heat through then add stock and water and bring to the boil.

2 Add spinach and simmer until cooked through. Add beans and stir through. Season with salt and pepper and add water to taste. Serve.

Serves 4–6

5-MINUTE DINNER PASTA

1 small red onion

1 clove garlic

2 tsp olive oil

1 small zucchini, cut into strips

2 roma tomatoes, chopped

210g can red salmon

4 asparagus spears

3 cups cooked pasta

¼ cup Parmesan cheese

1 Cook onion and garlic with olive oil in a frying pan over medium heat. Add zucchini and tomatoes and stir to heat through. Add salmon and cook for 1–2 minutes.

2 Add asparagus and cook for another minute. Mix through pasta, sprinkle with Parmesan and serve with a green salad.

Serves 4

SESAME CHICKEN

2 tbsp honey

2 tbsp sesame seeds

2 tbsp salt-reduced soy sauce

1 clove garlic, finely chopped

750g chicken breast, skin removed

1 tbsp sunflower oil

2 spring onions, finely chopped

2 cups broccoli florets, chopped into pieces

1 small red capsicum, finely chopped

2 cups cooked brown rice

1 Combine honey, sesame seeds, soy and garlic and set aside.

2 Cook chicken breast in frying pan over medium heat using a small amount of oil. Once chicken is cooked through, add honey and soy sauce with spring onions. Once heated through add broccoli and red capsicum and cook until broccoli is soft. Serve with brown rice.

Serves 4

SATAY ROO

500g kangaroo fillet

½ cup No Added Sugar Peanut Butter

1 tsp minced garlic

2 tsp minced chilli

Sprinkle of cumin and turmeric

2 sliced onions

1 Mix peanut butter, garlic, chilli and spices with warm water until pancake batter consistency is achieved.

2 Fry onions in wok, add kangaroo until lightly seared, then add sauce and warm until heated through.

3 Serve with salad.

Serves 2–4

CURRIED FISH

1 cup reduced-fat coconut milk

1 tbsp red or green curry paste

½ tsp brown sugar

juice of 1 lime

1 cup bok choy

4 x 180-200g white fish fillets

1 tsp light olive or canola oil

1 mushroom, sliced

1 cup sliced red capsicum

1 Simmer coconut milk, curry paste and brown sugar over a low heat until thickened. Add lime juice.

2 Lightly cook bok choy in a little water, set aside. Sear fish fillets in oil on skillet or frying pan until cooked through.

3 Remove fish and lightly cook vegetables on skillet.

4 Serve fish on bed of vegetables and drizzle with curry sauce.

Serves 4

Also works well with chicken breast or heaps of vegetables for the vegetarians.

HUMPDAY WEDNESDAY

The Wednesday plan

1. Take stock and remain mindful of what Wednesdays can mean.

2. Exert your control over alcohol.

3. Commit to one hard training session.

4. Get out and walk during the day.

5. Go light on Wednesday night.

✿ *Wednesdays can either make or break your diet commitment and weight loss outcomes.*

Take stock and remain mindful of what Wednesdays can mean

Once we make it through our Wednesday, things during the week are looking up. When it comes to weight loss, however, Wednesday can be the point in the week where things come undone. For this reason, remaining exceptionally mindful of our commitment, diet and exercise choices is imperative if we are to set up the second half of the week for successful weight loss. One way to ensure this happens is to always, at some point in the day, allow time to touch base with yourself and assess where things are up to from both an exercise and diet perspective.

Every Wednesday, allocate a 20–30 minute coffee or tea time-out when you can regroup and take stock of what needs to happen from this point in the week to ensure you are in control and on track. While things may not be 'perfect', or the way that you have intended them to be, taking a few minutes each Wednesday to regroup, take stock and make a plan to move forward is not only likely to be useful psychologically but also a way to see what needs to be done to keep your food and exercise on track come Thursday and Friday.

Exert your control over alcohol

❖ *Unfortunately, drinking too much, too often is the one thing that stands between you and weight loss.*

One particular issue that may arise on a Wednesday is the issue of drinking alcohol during the week, whether at home or when out socialising with friends, colleagues or family. Unfortunately, alcohol calories can really add up, and if you are serious about dropping weight and also being able to relax a little on the weekends, it is likely that you need a ban on alcohol during the week. The average alcoholic drink, whether it is beer, wine or spirits, contains as many calories as a slice of bread, and these calories will be preferentially burnt by the body before any food calories will. This means that in order to be losing weight while drinking alcohol three or more nights each week, you will need to be doing at least one hour of intense physical activity to burn off the alcohol calories as well as cutting down your caloric intake by at least 100–200 calories a day.

While eliminating alcohol during the week may be ideal, if it is not feasible or preferable, if you do enjoy a drink most nights and can limit yourself to just one alcoholic drink, as long as you also limit your meal size and carbohydrates you may still be able to achieve weight loss. This means that your dinner choices need to be a small portion of grilled lean red meat, chicken or fish with vegetables and avoiding all bread, rice, pasta and dessert, and, of course, watching the serving size of alcohol.

Commit to one hard training session

❧ *If you always think 'quality' over 'quantity' when it comes to exercise and metabolism, you will not go wrong.*

When the second half of the week rolls around, time is of the essence, which begs the question, why spend an hour at the gym or training when you can achieve the same caloric deficit by training hard for just 20–30 minutes? On Wednesdays, commit to a short, sharp interval-style training session where you burn at least 200–300 calories. Whether you achieve this via interval sprints, running hills, an intense session with a personal trainer or skipping, remember that the best thing you can do for your metabolic rate long term is to constantly challenge the cells to work harder, and you achieve this by really increasing your heart rate when training. For this reason, you are much better to go hard for a short period of time than walk or run for one hour or more.

❧ *If you consider that 20–30 minutes is just 2% of your day, no matter how busy you are you can find this time to train each Wednesday.*

Sample 30-minute training session

Hill sprints – 4 x 50 metres, 4 x 80 metres and 4 x 120 metres

Treadmill – hill incline, sprint for 30 seconds at 8–10 km/h then walk for 1 minute at 5–6 km/h and repeat

Skipping – 30 seconds on, 30 seconds off

Cycling – hard riding >100 rpm for 30 seconds then slow >60 rpm for 60 seconds

PT – mixed weights, skipping, sprinting as a circuit

Get out and walk during the day

It does not matter whether you take a stroll to run some errands or get changed and go for a workout or 30-minute power walk – just making sure that you use your Wednesday to move is crucial. Being relatively inactive during the day is known to be worse for our metabolism than anything we eat or drink, and breaking up the long working day is crucial as we try to work towards a better work/health/life balance.

Taking time out away from the desk gets your blood pumping, helps to clear glucose from the bloodstream and also clears your thoughts during a long working day. Remember that moving at lunchtime does not have to mean a full change into workout gear and a lot of sweating; it can simply mean a walk to get your lunch, some shopping to stock up on healthy snacks, running errands or meeting a friend for lunch. But the more movement you schedule into the day, the better.

One of the best ways to cement this commitment on Wednesdays is to do it with someone else. In the same way that you can team up with others to share a healthy lunch, so too can you commit to exercising with a buddy during your lunchbreak. Schedule a regular catch-up walk or lunch with a reliable colleague or friend so that it is cemented into your diary as any other appointment would be. Working hours are now commonly so long that we have to use our breaks and entitlements to look after our health, as we often simply do not have enough time left in our downtime to fit everything in.

Go light on Wednesday night

As the week progresses, Wednesday is often the last night before the fun part of the week is upon us. Unfortunately the 'fun' also tends to mean more calories thanks to more socialising and meals eaten away from home. For this reason, and as is the case for a strategy on Sunday nights, if you find yourself eating at home on a Wednesday night, choosing light meal options is a great way to help control your calorie intake a get ready for the next few days of higher calorie eating.

Going lighter on Wednesday may mean reducing your intake of rice, pasta, noodles and other carbohydrate-rich foods in favour of greater amounts of vegetables and lean protein. It could also mean swapping dinner for a soup or salad at times, especially if you know you have been eating more than you ideally should be, or if you have some big social events coming up over the next few days. It may also mean keeping your alcohol intake low, or eliminating it completely.

As a general rule of thumb, white fish and chicken breast are lighter protein options, as are tofu and shellfish. Just 100g of these protein choices, coupled with soup or salad, makes a perfect light 300 calorie dinner choice on Wednesday nights at home.

Wednesday snack list

4 corn crackers with 2 tbsp sugar-free peanut butter

Small skim coffee with 1 piece of biscotti

4 grain crackers with 40g cheese

½ cup mini tomatoes with 2 tbsp goats cheese

Mountain bread wrap with ham, cheese and tomato

WEDNESDAY VEGETABLE TIP:
Add a bowl of vegetable soup to your evening meal on Wednesdays to help keep your calorie intake at dinner low.

Wednesday meal plans

Breakfast
Ham and Cheese Toasty (page 123) OR ¾ cup (30g) bran cereal or 2 multigrain Weetbix with 1 cup low-fat milk with ½ cup berries or 2 kiwifruit

Lunch
Egg and Rocket Wrap (page 125) OR 1 wholegrain wrap with 2 eggs or 95g can tuna with 2 cups salad

Dinner
San Choy Bau (page 126) OR 2 cups beef or pork mince with 2 cups vegetables

Breakfast
Beans on Toast (page 123) OR small wholemeal wrap with 1 poached egg, 1 slice lean ham or bacon with rocket and 1 tbsp low-fat mayonnaise

Lunch
Asian Chicken Salad (page 125) OR ¼ BBQ chicken with small Greek salad

Dinner
Lamb Cutlets with Nuts and Vegetables (page 127) OR 100g grilled fillet steak/lean lamb fillet and large green salad

Breakfast
Breakfast Power Smoothie (page 123) OR meal replacement shake

Lunch
Lamb and Quinoa Salad (page 124) OR multigrain wrap with 100g chicken/turkey, 1 slice light Jarlsberg cheese, rocket and 1 tbsp cranberry sauce with ½ cup (125g) low-fat vanilla yoghurt

Dinner
Turkey Bolognaise (page 128) with 2 cups salad OR ½ cup cooked pasta with 10 prawns and 2 cups vegetables and tomato pasta sauce

Breakfast
Protein Pancakes (page 124) OR ¾ cup (30g) bran cereal or 1 multigrain Weetbix with 1 cup low-fat milk and ½ cup mixed berries

Lunch
Turkey Bolognaise (page 128) with ½ cup cooked pasta with 2 cups salad OR Salmon Triangle (page 126) with salad

Dinner
Sweet and Sour Pork (page 127) OR ½ cup cooked brown rice with 100g chicken or tuna, green beans, broccoli and snow peas with 2 tsp sweet chilli sauce

BEANS ON TOAST

½ cup or 130g can salt-reduced baked beans

1 slice grain bread, toasted

¼ avocado

1 slice light Jarlsberg cheese

Heat beans and serve on toast spread with thin layer of avocado and cheese slice.

Serves 1

BREAKFAST POWER SMOOTHIE

1 cup low-fat milk

2 heaped tbsp rolled oats

1 scoop caramel, vanilla or latte protein powder

2 tbsp natural low-fat yoghurt

1 tbsp LSA (ground linseed, sunflower seeds and almonds)

Add ice and blend.

Serves 1

HAM AND CHEESE TOASTY

2 slices sourdough or grain bread

1 tsp polyunsaturated fat spread

20g leg ham

1 slice reduced-fat cheese

⅓ cup cottage cheese

½ tomato, sliced

handful rocket leaves

Toast bread with small amount of spread, ham and cheeses. Slice and serve with tomato and rocket.

Serves 1

PROTEIN PANCAKES

1 egg

1 cup buttermilk

1 tbsp butter, softened

¾ cup plain flour

1 tsp baking powder

1 punnet berries

2 tbsp vanilla or berry protein powder

spray canola oil

ricotta cheese (optional)

1 Whisk together egg, buttermilk and butter. Add flour and baking powder and stir. Add berries and protein powder.

2 Add oil to frying pan and cook 2 tbsp batter over medium heat for 3 minutes on each side, until brown. Serve with a little ricotta if desired.

Serves 2

WEDNESDAY LUNCHES

LAMB AND QUINOA SALAD

4 vine-ripened tomatoes, sliced in half

1kg lamb back strap

2 tbsp olive oil

2 tbsp mint, finely chopped

2 tbsp flat-leaf parsley, finely chopped

1 x 400g can artichoke hearts, roughly chopped

2 cups cooked quinoa

50g Persian feta cheese, crumbled

1 Preheat oven to 150°C and roast tomatoes for 90 minutes.

2 Cook lamb over medium heat in a frying pan with a little olive oil for 5–7 minutes each side. Set aside to rest for 10 minutes before slicing.

3 Stir herbs and artichoke through quinoa with 1 tbsp olive oil. Sprinkle with feta.

4 Serve sliced lamb and tomatoes with salad.

Serves 4

ASIAN CHICKEN SALAD

2 tbsp sunflower oil

¼ cup lime juice

pinch of salt

4 cups mixed lettuce leaves

2–3 cups shredded BBQ chicken

¼ red cabbage

1 red capsicum, finely sliced

½ cup cashew nuts

1 Combine oil and lime juice with a little salt and set aside.

2 Combine remaining ingredients and drizzle with lime and oil dressing.

Serves 2

EGG AND ROCKET WRAPS

2 hard-boiled eggs

1 tbsp reduced-fat egg mayonnaise

2 tsp pesto

2 wholegrain wraps

1 cup rocket leaves

2 tsp sweet chilli sauce

1 Mash eggs with mayonnaise and pesto.

2 Spread egg mixture on wrap and top with rocket and a drizzle of sweet chilli sauce.

Serves 2

SALMON TRIANGLES

2 spring onions, sliced

1 red capsicum, chopped finely

1 tbsp butter

2 tbsp flour

¼ cup low-fat milk

¼ cup reduced-fat cream

415g can red salmon

4–6 sheets filo pastry

olive oil spray

baby spinach leaves

1 Cook onion and capsicum in butter in a saucepan over medium heat. Add flour and once mixture bubbles, add milk and cream and stir until slightly thickened.

2 Remove from heat and stir in salmon.

3 Spray filo sheets with olive oil and add salmon mixture, folding to make 6–8 triangles.

4 Bake for 5–10 minutes, until pastry is golden. Serve with salad.

Serves 4

WEDNESDAY DINNERS

SAN CHOY BAU

1 brown onion, finely chopped

1 tsp crushed garlic

1 tbsp olive oil

1 small chilli, chopped

500g extra lean beef mince

2 carrots, finely chopped

2 sticks celery, finely chopped

8 button mushrooms, finely sliced

4 tbsp salt-reduced soy sauce

8 large lettuce leaves

1 Fry onion and garlic in olive oil until soft. Add chilli and beef and cook until browned.

2 Add vegetables and soy sauce and continue cooking until beef is cooked through.

3 Serve in lettuce cups.

Serves 4–6

SWEET AND SOUR PORK

1 tbsp cornflour
¼ cup sugar
1 tbsp salt-reduced soy sauce
¼ cup white vinegar
1 tbsp sunflower oil
1kg lean pork fillet
2 cups green beans
1 green capsicum, finely sliced
1 red capsicum, finely sliced
2 spring onions, finely chopped
2 garlic cloves, finely chopped
¼ cup raw almonds
1 cup cooked brown rice (optional)

1 Whisk together cornflour, sugar, soy sauce and vinegar and set aside.

2 Heat oil in a hot frying pan. Add pork and stir until cooked through. Add beans and capsicum and cook until vegetables begin to soften. Add spring onion and garlic and cook for a further 3–5 minutes.

3 Add soy sauce mixture and cook until sauce thickens. Add almonds and stir to heat through. Serve with brown rice if desired.

Serves 4

LAMB CUTLETS WITH NUTS AND VEGETABLES

olive or canola oil spray
8 lean lamb cutlets
150g (1 punnet) grape tomatoes
1 cup quartered artichoke hearts
1 red capsicum, diced
1 cup corn kernels
⅓ cup shelled pistachios, finely chopped
2 tsp olive oil
50g Danish feta, crumbled

1 Using spray oil, cook lamb cutlets in a large frying pan over medium heat until browned.

2 Add vegetables to one-half of the pan, along with pistachios and olive oil.

3 Once tomatoes are cooked through, remove vegetables from pan, sprinkle with feta and serve with cutlets.

Serves 4

TURKEY BOLOGNAISE

1 large onion, finely diced

2 cloves garlic, finely diced

1 tbsp olive oil

1 large carrot, finely diced

2 sticks celery, finely chopped

500g turkey mince

¼ cup white wine

3 tbsp salt-reduced tomato paste

400g can diced tomatoes

1 cup salt-reduced chicken stock

2 cups penne pasta, boiled (optional)

1 Cook onion and garlic with olive oil until translucent. Add carrot and celery and cook for a further 5 minutes. Add turkey mince and cook until browned.

2 Add wine and cook until wine has evaporated. Add tomato paste and tomatoes and cook for a further 10 minutes.

3 Add chicken stock and simmer over medium heat for 30–60 minutes. Serve with cooked penne if desired.

Serves 4

FUNDAY THURSDAY

The Thursday plan

1. Log your calories.

2. Compensate when you overdo things.

3. Book in training.

4. Weigh in.

5. Grab a protein-rich snack late afternoon.

❂ *Thursdays are just like Tuesdays but can be the day*
in which we lose our focus.

Log your calories

One of the biggest dietary issues associated with the days in the second half of the week is that not only do we eat extra calories but we often have a complete calorie blowout, eating foods that we never usually would, and in large amounts. While consuming an extra 200–300 calories in a single meal is unlikely to cause any long-term issues with weight control, if we are regularly consuming 500–600 more calories in a single meal, then weight control, let alone weight loss, is going to be exceptionally challenging. While it may sound difficult to consume this many extra calories, if you consider that a single piece of cake or dessert or a 2- or 3-course meal will easily give you this many extra calories, it becomes clear how easy it is to overeat.

As the end of the week rolls around, and eating out becomes a more frequent occurrence, self-monitoring your calories via an online monitoring program such as 'myfitnesspal' is a good way to gain insight into exactly how many extra calories you may be consuming when you eat out, and also whether you need to compensate with a lighter meal when you have overdone things.

As mentioned, an extra 200–300 calories that come from enjoying dessert or an extra course is not the end of the world, but if you are enjoying an extra 500 or even 1000 calories from wine, bread, heavy food choices and dessert, and you dine out more than once a fortnight, you may need to pull things back a little.

❂ *The average female wanting to lose weight will*
need just 1200 calories each day, while a male
needs just 1600–1800 calories.

Compensate when you overdo things

One of the most powerful steps you can take towards weight control long term is to learn to compensate when you have overdone things: have a light meal if you have had a heavy one, skip a snack if you are not hungry, or put in extra gym time to compensate when you have eaten too much. Often a period of chronic overconsumption gives way to continual overeating as we become used to eating more and more food and forget just how little we really need.

Restaurant and fast-food serves do nothing to help with this, with the average meal we enjoy away from home containing at least 25–30% more calories than the meals we would prepare for ourselves at home. This means that if you do not feel like dinner after a big lunch, or a large breakfast after a night out, there is no need to eat when you are not hungry. In fact, a light meal or skipping a meal altogether is likely to be just what you need to get your body and appetite back on track.

An easy way to actively compensate when you have eaten out, and a way that will also benefit your metabolism, is to factor in extra activity to compensate when you have enjoyed extra calories. Walk home, do an extra gym class or personal trainer session, particularly at times when you have a number of extra social occasions. Not only will your digestion benefit but your weight is at least likely to be stable rather than increase.

❧ *The art of compensating when you have over-consumed calories is an easy way to ensure that eating out does not have to negatively affect your weight.*

Book in training

It is natural to need a little push sometimes when it comes to exercise, even for the most motivated among us, especially as the end of the week rolls around. As Thursday and Friday nights are often when we enjoy eating out, it makes sense to commit to training on a Thursday every week and even better sense to actually make these the sessions that are booked in with a friend, trainer or set class.

Humans respond exceptionally well to rules and structure, and this means that when it comes to training, the more regulated we are the better. Earlier in the week it tends to be easier to get to the gym or fit in an early-morning walk or run, whereas by Thursday we are tired and need that extra incentive. When you consider that Thursday tends to be the time in the week when things start to go off track, it makes sense to commit to a high-intensity training session each and every Thursday.

Intensity is everything when it comes to getting the most out of your training, especially if you are already relatively fit and your focus is on weight loss. While you may only be able to dedicate 20 or 30 minutes to training on a Thursday, make the 20 or 30 minutes really count – run intervals or hills, alternate between gym machines, or increase your weights or the intensity of the gym machine. As a general rule of thumb, aiming to burn 100 calories every 10 minutes that you train is a good marker of high-intensity, metabolically beneficial, cardio-style training.

Weigh in

If there is one piece of information that is likely to be motivating when it comes to keeping on track with your diet, it is knowing whether your weight is dropping, stable or, heaven forbid, creeping up. Weighing in on a regular basis is one of the most powerful things you can do to keep your weight under control, and there is no better day of the week to do this than on a Thursday. It is long enough after the weekend to have recovered from any sins, but perfect timing to remind you to keep focused over the upcoming weekend.

To keep on track on your Thursday, and ultimately for the days ahead, set aside time to weigh yourself first thing in the morning. Keeping a close eye on your body weight not only reminds you to take each and every food decision that you make on a daily basis seriously, but it is also a great way to remind you that even though the weekend is nigh, your hard work for the past 4 days cannot be completely discarded. Taking your weight will give an indication of how much you can indulge over the weekend while helping to keep you focused on your long-term goals.

Grab a protein-rich snack late afternoon

One of the secrets to keeping your diet on track, even though you may eat out regularly, is to never put yourself in the position where you arrive at a function, dinner or bar when you are hungry. Making food or menu selections when you are hungry means that you are more likely to order and eat more than you usually would, which for those of us who eat out regularly can be a significant barrier between achieving weight-loss results and not.

The easiest way to manage this is to schedule a protein-rich snack — such as a shake, bar, serve of nuts or cottage cheese — an hour or two before you leave for your event. This strategy works particularly well as the end of the week draws near and Thursday or Friday drinks or social outings become more common. Such a strategy works well even if you are just going shopping after work or have to run around after the kids, taking them to sports practice or school events. It is the times when we become extremely hungry, as often occurs late in the afternoon, that we seek out quick hits of high-calorie, sweet-tasting foods. Once you prevent this craving using protein–rich foods, you will find that you no longer experience the energy drop come 5 or 6pm and can remain in control of your appetite and your food choices.

For some, especially workers who spend 10–12 hours each day at work, scheduling a late-afternoon snack may also mean that you are eating both an afternoon tea and then another snack before you leave work. While this may seem to be a lot of extra food, the benefit of keeping on top of your appetite outweighs the issue of consuming an extra 100–200 calories.

Late Thursday pre-event snacks

Low-carb protein bar

Meal replacement shake

2 corn crackers with cottage cheese

30g almonds with 20g cheese

100g Greek-style yoghurt with 1 tsp protein powder

Thursday snack list

4 rye crackers with light cream cheese and tomato

Small skim milk coffee with 20g dark chocolate

20g cheese with 2 cups popcorn

Low-carb protein bar

1 slice grain toast with 1tbsp cottage cheese and cucumber

THURSDAY VEGETABLE TIP:
Keep celery and cucumber on hand to munch on during the day to help reduce bloating and prevent overeating.

Thursday exercise ideas

1. Schedule a weekly stretch, yoga or pilates class to keep active.

2. Walk to dinner or drinks.

3. Get off the bus or train a stop or two earlier.

4. Walk home from dinner or go for a family walk after you eat.

5. Join a local Zumba or dance class.

Thursday meal plans

Breakfast
Breakfast Cereal Mix (page 136) OR ¾ cup bran or oat cereal with 200ml natural yoghurt with 1 tsp cinnamon and ½ cup berries

Lunch

Chicken and Tomato Salad (page 139) OR 2 California sushi rolls with seaweed salad and miso soup

Dinner

Steak and Potatoes (page 141) OR 100g lean steak fillet with ½ corn cob, roasted pumpkin and mixed green salad

Breakfast

Veggie Scramble (page 137) OR 1 slice wholegrain toast with ½ cup baked beans with 1 small glass (200ml) vegetable juice

Lunch

Asian Salmon Salad (page 138) OR Steak Salad (page 138)

Dinner

100g grilled chicken breast with 1 cup of mashed pumpkin and 1 cup of snow peas and green beans

Breakfast

Fruit Salad and Yoghurt (page 136) OR low-fat milk berry smoothie with 1 tsp protein powder

Lunch

Quinoa Patties (page 139) with 2 cups salad OR turkey and salad wholegrain wrap

Dinner

5-Minute Prawn Stir Fry (page 141) OR 100g chicken fillet or 10 green prawns stir fried with carrots, red capsicum, snow peas and broccoli in 2 tbsp oyster sauce, and ½ cup cooked brown rice

Breakfast
Ricotta Honey Wrap (page 137) OR 1 slice wholegrain toast with
⅓ cup cottage cheese with sliced tomato and 1 piece fruit

Lunch
Stuffed Potato OR ½ cup cooked brown rice with 95g can tuna
and 1 cup mixed vegetables with 1 tsp sweet chilli sauce OR Warm
Lamb Salad (page 140)

Dinner
Quick Veggie Pot (page 140) OR stir fried vegetables and tofu
without rice

THURSDAY BREAKFASTS

BREAKFAST CEREAL MIX

⅓ cup rolled oats or bran cereal

200g natural yoghurt

2 tsp vanilla protein powder

½ cup berries

2–3 drops vanilla essence

Mix all ingredients together and place in a glass or bowl to serve.

Serves 1

FRUIT SALAD AND YOGHURT

1 cup mixed chopped fruit

1 cup Greek-style yoghurt

2 tsp chia seeds

Top the fruit with yoghurt and sprinkle with chia seeds.

Serves 1

VEGGIE SCRAMBLE

olive oil spray

½ Spanish onion, finely chopped

1 tomato, diced

30g mushrooms, sliced

2 free-range eggs, lightly beaten

30g low-fat tasty cheese, grated

20g lean ham, diced

1 Place a non-stick frying pan over medium heat and spray lightly with oil.

2 Add the onion, tomato and mushrooms and cook for about 1 minute, until translucent. Move the vegetables to one side of the pan and add the beaten egg.

3 While the egg is cooking, add the cheese and ham to the vegetables. Once the scramble is almost set, fold over the top of the vegetables and serve.

Serves 1

RICOTTA HONEY WRAPS

¼ cup low-fat ricotta

½ cup Greek-style yoghurt

2 tsp honey

2 wholegrain wraps

1 green apple, finely sliced

1 Combine ricotta, yoghurt and honey.

2 Spread mixture over half the wrap and top with ½ sliced apple. Roll and serve.

Serves 2

ASIAN SALMON SALAD

200g salmon fillet

4 cups mixed lettuce leaves

1 cup finely sliced red capsicum

1 cup grated carrot

½ cup cashew nuts

1 tbsp sesame oil

½ lime

1 Grill salmon and flake through lettuce leaves. Add capsicum, carrot and cashew nuts.

2 Dress with sesame oil and lime juice. Serve.

Serves 2

STEAK SALAD

200g rib-eye or rump steak

1 tbsp olive oil

1 tbsp Dijon mustard

2 cups sugar snap peas

4 cups mixed lettuce leaves

8 radishes, sliced

2 carrots, grated

1 red capsicum, finely sliced

1 Grill steak and cut into slices. Mix olive oil and mustard together.

2 Lightly steam snap peas.

3 Mix all salad ingredients and top with Dijon mustard dressing.

Serves 2

CHICKEN AND TOMATO SALAD

500g lean chicken breast
fillets

4 sticks celery, finely chopped

2 Lebanese cucumbers, finely
chopped

1 cup chick peas, rinsed

1 cup grape tomatoes, sliced

4 tbsp pesto

½ lemon

1 Grill chicken fillets and cut into slices.

2 Place salad ingredients in a bowl. Add chicken and dress with pesto and a squeeze of lemon juice. Serve.

Serves 4

QUINOA PATTIES

2½ cups cooked quinoa

4 large eggs, beaten

6 cloves garlic, crushed

⅔ cup chopped fresh chives

1 red onion, finely chopped

⅓ cup freshly grated
Parmesan cheese

1 cup wholegrain
breadcrumbs

extra virgin olive oil spray

1 Combine quinoa and beaten egg. Stir in garlic, chives, onion and Parmesan cheese.

2 Add breadcrumbs and form into 6cm patties. The mixture should be very moist.

3 Place a frying pan over medium heat and spray with olive oil. Cover and cook patties for 8–10 minutes, until brown. Flip and cook for another 7 minutes on the other side. Serve with a large salad.

Serves 2–3

WARM LAMB SALAD

3–4 cups of assorted lettuce leaves

1 Lebanese cucumber, roughly chopped

1 medium red capsicum, seeded and sliced

4 roma tomatoes, roughly chopped

200g sweet potato, diced and roasted

50g reduced-fat feta cheese, crumbled

200g lean lamb fillets

1 tbsp olive oil

tzatziki yoghurt dip

1 Combine lettuce, vegetables and feta cheese in a bowl.

2 Massage lamb fillets with olive oil. Sear lightly in a very hot wok or frying pan until medium–rare. Rest for 5–10 minutes then slice into thin pieces.

3 Add lamb to salad and dress with tzatziki.

Serves 2

THURSDAY DINNERS

VEGGIE HOT POT

1 tbsp olive oil

1 medium onion, finely chopped

2 garlic cloves, finely chopped

1 large zucchini, finely chopped

1 green capsicum, finely sliced

1 tbsp chilli powder

1 tsp ground cumin

420g can corn kernels

420g can red kidney beans

400g can crushed tomatoes

¼ cup reduced-fat sour cream

1 Heat olive oil in a large saucepan and cook onion and garlic until translucent. Add zucchini, capsicum, chilli powder and cumin and cook for 10–15 minutes over medium heat until vegetables are tender.

2 Add corn, beans, tomatoes and 1 cup water. Simmer until soft and serve with a dollop of sour cream.

Serves 4

5-MINUTE PRAWN STIR FRY

2 small red chillies, finely chopped

1 tbsp olive oil

2 cloves garlic, crushed

1 onion, finely sliced

40 green prawns

1 red capsicum, finely sliced

1 carrot, chopped

1 cup green beans, prepared

1 cup broccoli florets

4 tbsp sweet chilli sauce

250g flat rice noodles, cooked

handful fresh basil leaves

1 Stir-fry chilli, olive oil, garlic and onion over high heat until onion is translucent.

2 Add prawns and cook until pink.

3 Add vegetables, sweet chilli sauce and rice noodles and heat through.

4 Add basil leaves and serve.

Serves 4

STEAK AND POTATOES

2 x 200g beef fillet steaks

1 cup green beans, steamed

1 cup carrots, sliced, steamed

2 medium jacket potatoes, baked

1 Sear steak over medium heat until cooked to liking.

2 Serve with steamed vegetables and a jacket potato.

Serves 2

TGI FRIDAY

The Friday plan

1. Relax a little.

2. Keep on track until lunchtime.

3. Enjoy lunch out.

4. Be smart at drinks.

5. Get rid of the 'all or nothing' approach.

❁ *Fridays mean fun and the weekend, but they can also mean a major calorie blowout if we are not careful.*

Relax a little

One of the best things about keeping your diet and training strict for most of the week is that you get a little more freedom come the weekend. While this does not mean letting things go completely off track, it does mean that if you want to enjoy lunch out or a couple of drinks after work, the progress you have made thus far will not be completely disrupted. The trick is to learn over time how to let things go a little: to learn the skills that will help you have 2 or 3 drinks instead of 10; to have one meal off for a special occasion, not 2–3 days of poor eating; to skip one training session, not 2 weeks of training. For some, this is an easy skill to adopt and put into practice – in fact many of us have learnt how to do this from parents and mentors when we were small. For others, acquiring this skill is far more challenging and it takes constant effort to practise and reinforce before it becomes second nature.

At times there will be particularly special occasions in which you really let things go. But more commonly, our Fridays are simply another day in the week in which we need to learn to manage our food and drinking behaviours so we can indeed have a good time but without blowing our calories out the window completely, simply because it is Friday.

❖ *Before you head out on a Friday night, decide how many drinks you will indulge in and stick to your limit.*

Keep on track until lunchtime

If you begin the day with banana bread, a muffin or any less than ideal breakfast, it is safe to say that things will go downhill nutritionally from there. Make it a priority to enjoy a breakfast that contains some sort of protein, even on Fridays. While it may be something heavier, such as a lean bacon and egg sandwich, omelette or other store bought breakfast, concentrate on protein-rich choices to help keep your appetite under control throughout the morning. Alternatively, you may find that swapping your breakfast to a shake or other low-calorie option is a good way to compensate if you know that you always enjoy lunch out on Fridays.

❖ *We do not gain weight because we enjoy a single meal or night out; we gain weight when we take an entire day off our diet plan.*

Enjoy lunch out

Whether it is a social occasion or office ritual, eating lunch out on a Friday is a weekly tradition and, as is the case with any meal you do not prepare for yourself, it all comes down to knowing what to choose from the menu. The good news about eating out, particularly in the city, is that in general there are reasonably good options and the real issue is whether you choose these or not. As a general rule of thumb, anything fried – from noodles, fish, chips and fast food from chain-style eateries – is never going to be a great choice. These are generally lacking in nutrition, high in fat and easily over-consumed thanks to their soft, sludgy nature.

Instead, if you simply look for options on a menu that contain protein – fish, chicken, steak, egg in some form, whether it be in a burger, stir fry, fish meal or wrap – you will be on the right track. If you can add some sort of salad or vegetables, even better. While a steak sandwich or chicken schnitzel may be relatively high in fat compared to your regular lunch, at least they contain a good source of protein and, ideally, salad or vegetables – unlike pasta, risottos, fried fish and chips or pies, which contain much fat but little else nutritionally.

When it comes to long lunches, the same rules apply. Think seafood, vegetables and lean protein and you will not go wrong. Another trick is to have a small snack such as a protein shake or bar before you head out for a long lunch, so you are not so hungry and therefore in a position to make better food choices.

❧ *No matter where you are, or what you are eating, always make sure your lunch contains some vegetables and/or salad.*

Be smart at drinks

It is Friday afternoon and you have had a big week and worked hard. Of course there is nothing wrong with letting off a little steam after work and enjoying a few drinks and relaxation time with your colleagues. Before you head out, always have a clear idea in your mind of how many drinks you plan to have. When you make this decision before heading out, it is much easier to say no once you reach your limit. Choose clear spirits with low-calorie mixers over wine and beer because they contain fewer calories, and look for snacks and bar food that are not fried.

❧ *Never head out to drinks hungry or you will be sure to overeat. Always keep a protein-rich snack to grab an hour or two before you leave for your function.*

Get rid of the 'all or nothing' approach

Yes, you have made it through another week, and yes, that is grounds to celebrate, albeit on a small scale. But before you overdo it, here are a couple of things to consider. Many of us have so many social and family commitments scheduled during our precious two-day weekend that blowing it all for a big Friday night on the town or a calorie fest in front of the television really seems like a waste, doesn't it?

The best thing you can do on a Friday night is either have a great night out with people you love, rather than work colleagues you barely know, or spend quality time at home with family, taking time to relax and unwind in preparation for a great weekend. Take time to prepare a tasty yet healthy version of your favourite pizza or 'fun' family meal, clean up so that you do not have to do it over the weekend, and get an early night so you greet your Saturday feeling refreshed and focused.

Friday snack list

100g fruit yoghurt

30g mixed nuts and small punnet of berries

Small skim milk coffee

1 apple/pear and 20g cheese

2 corn crackers with ¼ cup cottage cheese/goat's cheese and tomato

FRIDAY VEGETABLE TIP:

Grab a cup of soup an hour or two before work finishes to take the edge off your hunger before you head out.

Friday exercise ideas

1. Start the day with a quick training session to get it out of the way.

2. Walk to work or walk home.

3. Schedule a work bonding training session.

4. Meet your partner for dinner and walk to the restaurant together.

5. Schedule a late Friday afternoon stretch or relaxation class to ease you into the weekend.

Friday meal plans

Breakfast
Protein Slice (page 148) OR 2 slices multigrain toast with ¼ avocado and tomato

Lunch
Thai Beef Salad with Chilli Dressing (page 151) with 1 piece of fruit OR Chicken Greek Salad

Dinner
Sausages and Veggie Mash (page 152) OR 2 lean sausages with mashed pumpkin, potato and peas

Breakfast
Quick Bacon Wrap (page 149) OR wholemeal bacon and egg roll without butter

Lunch
Lighter Quiche (page 150) with 2 cups salad OR a turkey or chicken wrap

Dinner
5-Minute Pizza (page 152) with 2 cups salad OR 2 slices thin crust pizza with large side salad

Breakfast
Mini Bircher (page 149) OR ¾ cup (30g) bran cereal or 1 multi-grain Weetbix with 1 cup low-fat milk and 1 piece of fruit

Lunch
Chicken and Apple Salad (page 150) OR ¾ cup cooked brown rice or pasta with 100g chicken breast with sweet chilli sauce and mixed green salad

Dinner
Healthy Fish and Chips (page 153) OR 150g grilled white fish with Greek salad

Breakfast

Cheese and Salmon on Crackers (page 149) OR bacon or smoked salmon and rocket wrap

Lunch

Steak sandwich on grain bread OR 2 California sushi rolls with 250ml mixed vegetable juice

Dinner

Tuna Mac and Cheese (page 153) with 2 cups salad OR entree-sized serve spaghetti marinara with salad

FRIDAY BREAKFASTS

PROTEIN SLICE

1 cup (160g) vanilla protein powder

2 cups rolled oats

2 tsp cinnamon

2 eggs

2 tbsp butter

2 tsp honey

½ cup skim milk

1 Preheat oven to 180°C. Mix protein powder, oats and cinnamon in a bowl. Add remaining ingredients and mix until well combined.

2 Pour into greased baking dish and bake for 15–20 minutes, until firm.

Serves 6–8

QUICK BACON WRAP

50g lean bacon

olive oil spray

½ tomato, sliced

1 cup rocket leaves

1 tbsp mayonnaise

1 tsp sweet chilli or tomato sauce

1 wholegrain wrap

Fry bacon with a little spray oil. Combine with remaining ingredients on a wholegrain wrap.

Serves 1

CHEESE AND SALMON ON CRACKERS

4 corn or rice cakes

½ cup cottage or goat's cheese

50g smoked salmon

few sprigs dill

Spread crackers with cheese and top with smoked salmon. Garnish with dill and serve.

Serves 1

MINI BIRCHER

¼ cup rolled oats

½ cup reduced-fat milk

150g natural Greek-style yoghurt

½ cup berries

1 tsp honey

1 Soak oats in milk overnight.

2 Stir in yoghurt and serve with berries and a drizzle of honey.

Serves 1

CHICKEN AND APPLE SALAD

¼ cup buttermilk

2 tbsp mayonnaise

1 tbsp white wine vinegar

200g chicken breast fillets, grilled

4 cups mixed lettuce leaves

1 Pink Lady apple, cut into wedges

½ cup dried cranberries

2 slices crusty Italian bread

1 Combine buttermilk, mayonnaise and vinegar and set aside.

2 Slice chicken and mix with lettuce leaves, apple and cranberries. Drizzle with a little dressing and serve with bread.

Serves 2

LIGHTER QUICHE

4 eggs

1½ cups low-fat milk

½ cup self-raising flour

3 tbsp melted butter or margarine

1½ cups grated low-fat cheese

2 cups of filling of your choice (red salmon, chopped tomatoes, corn, capsicum, English spinach leaves, grated zucchini or carrot, sliced mushrooms, onion, ham or leftover BBQ chicken)

olive oil spray

1 Preheat oven to 180°C. Whisk together the eggs, milk, flour and butter.

2 Fold through the cheese and the fillings.

3 Spray an overproof dish lightly with olive oil, pour mixture in and bake for 40 minutes.

4 Serve with a side salad.

Serves 6

THAI BEEF SALAD WITH CHILLI DRESSING

1 garlic clove, finely chopped

1 coriander root, finely chopped

1 tbsp olive oil

100g rump or sirloin steak

150g soft lettuce, washed and roughly torn into pieces

100g cherry tomatoes, halved

75g cucumber, sliced

2 tbsp spring onion, finely chopped

1 tbsp coriander leaves, chopped

Chilli dressing

1 tbsp Thai fish sauce

1 tbsp lime juice

1 tbsp salt-reduced soy sauce

1 tbsp finely chopped red chilli

1   Combine the garlic, coriander root, black pepper and half the oil in a mortar and pound with a pestle until fine (or use a food processor or blender). Spread the mixture over the steak.

2   Heat the remaining oil in a heavy-based frying pan or wok over high heat. Cook the steak for 4 minutes on each side, turning once. Remove and set aside to cool.

3   Arrange lettuce, tomatoes, cucumber and spring onion on a plate.

4   Mix together the dressing ingredients.

5   Cut the cooled steak into thin strips and arrange on top of the salad. Drizzle over the dressing, scatter with coriander leaves and serve.

Serves 1

SAUSAGES AND VEGGIE MASH

8 lean (<10% fat) sausages

1 onion, finely sliced

1 small garlic clove, crushed

olive oil spray

1 zucchini, grated

1 large carrot, grated

1 small butternut pumpkin, diced and pre-cooked in microwave

¼ cup extra-light sour cream

2 tsp wholegrain mustard

1 Grill sausages until cooked through.

2 In a frying pan, sauté onion and garlic over olive oil. Add zucchini and carrot and cook through. Remove and mash all vegetables together.

3 Mix sour cream and mustard together and serve mash with a little sour cream drizzle.

Serves 4

5-MINUTE PIZZA

1 slice oat or wholewheat Mountain Bread

1 tbsp salt-reduced tomato paste

50g 97% fat-free ham or chicken breast fillet, sliced

handful baby spinach leaves

50g feta cheese, crumbled

30g reduced-fat tasty cheese, grated

1 Preheat oven to 200°C.

2 Cover the bread with a thin layer of tomato paste. Top with ham, spinach leaves and cheeses.

3 Bake for 10 minutes, or until the cheese has melted.

4 Serve with salad.

Serves 1

HEALTHY FISH AND CHIPS

200g sweet potato, cut into wedges

olive oil spray

2 cups cornflakes, crushed

1 egg, beaten

2 tbsp low-fat natural yoghurt

600g boneless white fish fillets

½ cup wholemeal flour

1 Preheat oven to 190°C. Dry bake sweet potato at 180°C for 30–40 minutes until brown and crispy.

2 Put cornflakes on a plate. Combine egg and yoghurt in a bowl. Dip fish in flour then the egg mixture and then coat with cornflakes.

3 Place fish on a separate baking tray and bake at 180°C for 15–20 minutes or until crumb is crisp and brown.

Serves 4

TUNA MAC AND CHEESE

1 tbsp butter

1 tbsp plain flour

1 cup low-fat milk

¼ cup carrot, grated

¼ cup zucchini, grated

¼ cup corn kernels

2 x 95g cans 97% fat-free tuna

1 cup cooked macaroni

½ cup light cheddar cheese, grated

1 Heat butter in a saucepan over medium heat, add flour and cook, stirring, for 1 minute.

2 Remove pan from the heat and stir in the milk. Return to the heat and cook, stirring, until the sauce boils and thickens.

3 Add vegetables, tuna and macaroni and cook for 5 minutes, or until vegetables are soft. Stir in the cheese and cook until it has melted. Serve with salad.

Serves 2

How to get back on track when things fall off the rails or 'the quick reset'

✼ *I know what I should be eating, but sometimes life takes over and I find myself back where I started.*

One of the key skills of individuals who control their weight is that they rarely have times when things go completely off the rails. Sure, they may have one heavier meal occasionally or skip the gym a few days in a row, but ultimately their baseline health habits are so deeply entrenched that they always return to a strong routine of eating well most of the time and exercising a certain number of times each week.

Some of us find this a little more difficult, and a few detours from our normal routine can quickly see us return to our less-than-ideal lifestyle habits. The secret to shifting this behavioural pattern is to become more aware of the times when you find yourself off track and develop contingency plans to manage the situation. So, if you know that it has been several days since you have exercised, schedule it in for the next day rather than waiting again until the following Monday to get started. Or take control of your food by making a soup or salad that night to get back on track the next day. Rather than ruminating on what you *should* be doing, start to just 'do' it – whether it is going for a walk, cooking or going to bed so you can get up early and make it to the gym the next day.

For times when you have gone off track and need to cut the calories for a couple of days in order to drop some weight quickly, you can either return to the Reset Monday or follow a light calorie intake, such as the one below, for 2–3 days to get you back on track physically and mentally. There is no issue with following a low-calorie eating plan for a few days, but remember that after 2–3 days you will need to consume more nutrients and calories and return to your regular, nutritionally balanced food plans.

The Quick Reset Plan

DAY 1	FOOD
Breakfast	2 tbsp bran + 1 cup fruit salad + 2 tbsp natural yoghurt
Snack	Cup of green tea + 2 rye crackers + 2 tbsp cottage cheese
Lunch	95g can tuna/salmon + mixed salad + 130g can corn + 1 tsp olive oil
Mid-Afternoon	15 mixed nuts + mandarin
Dinner	100g chicken breast + stir fried green vegetables in 1 tsp olive oil

DAY 2	FOOD
Breakfast	1 egg omelette with 1 cup chopped veggies (mushrooms, tomatoes, capsicum)
Midmorning	Small skim coffee
Lunch	4 rye crackers + 95g can tuna/salmon + mixed salad + 1 piece of fruit
Midafternoon	½ cup Greek-style yoghurt + 15 nuts
Dinner	100g salmon, roast pumpkin + mixed salad

DAY 3	FOOD
Breakfast	Protein shake with 200ml skim milk with 1 tsp protein
Midmorning	½ cup low-fat yoghurt + 1 piece of fruit
Lunch	Bowl of vegetable soup + 2 rye crackers + ¼ avocado
Midafternoon	Cut up vegetable sticks ½ cup low-fat hummus
Dinner	100g white fish + bowl of vegetable soup

What about alcohol?

❖ *To drink or not to drink during the week, now that is the question.*

In an ideal world we could get home after a big day, pour a glass of classic Pinot Noir or our favourite Sauvignon Blanc and mindfully sip one small glass before moving on to dinner. Unfortunately, in real life the scenario looks something like this: you just make it in the door weighted down with schoolbags, work stuff, gym clothes and a tennis racket and stumble over to the fridge to pour yourself a large glass of any alcoholic beverage you can find. Then you proceed to drink the rest of the bottle in front of the television as you lie there, broken and exhausted. Or you have after-work drinks where colleagues encourage you to consume numerous drinks as a way of blotting out the reality of life.

There is nothing wrong with enjoying a drink, but more often than not we enjoy too many drinks, and far too often. The issue with this level of consumption is that alcohol contains a significant number of calories. But the bigger issue is the fact that we tend to become completely disinhibited as we drink. This means that paying attention to what we eat, do or say while we are drinking has no boundaries. We eat far more of the wrong types of food than we usually would when we are drinking, and any chance of exercising or completing tasks and fulfilling activities at home becomes less and less likely.

Enjoying a few drinks on the weekend poses no issue – you work hard and if you find that a couple of beers or glasses of wine helps you relax and enjoy your down time, so be it. Too often, however, a few drinks becomes a complete binge and an entire day or two is wasted due to the effects of alcohol. Again, this is a personal choice, but if it is a weekly occurrence then it might be worth considering if it is really worth wasting so much of your precious time dealing with the long-term effects of alcohol abuse.

When it comes to cutting back on how much you are drinking during the week, the truth is that few of us can drink regularly and not experience some weight side effects as a result. For this reason, developing your own rules when it comes to drinking during the week is a good way to work towards balance in your drinking and your weight. This will mean having a number of alcohol-free days during the week or sticking to just half to a single glass of wine each day. Everyone will have a different preference in the way they decide to self-manage their alcohol intake.

If you do regularly arrive home from work and find yourself pouring a drink as soon as you walk in the door, it may be worth taking some time to consider the real reason why you are drinking. Do you actually enjoy it, or is it more a mindless habit that you have developed over time? Once drinking becomes a habit, it can become so entrenched in your lifestyle that it can become a very difficult habit to break, and what was once a single glass of wine is more likely to be half a bottle every single day. The result is that your evenings become unproductive and you sleep badly and wake in the mornings feeling fatigued and slightly hung-over. So, if you are a nightly drinker and finding that the habit is starting to nega-tively impact on your life in numerous ways, it may really be time to take a break from drinking altogether. It is only when you have completely removed yourself from something that you have the mental clarity to see the effect it is having on your life. Only then can you make an informed decision over what role alcohol should play in your week.

One thing to be mindful of when considering how much you should be drinking is to consider whether you are drinking socially or because of your work. Professionals can regularly find themselves at work functions where it seems that everyone is drinking. Whether it is an after-work drinks gathering, a lunchtime function or conference, the pressure to drink comes from all angles: in order to 'fit in', to be enjoying yourself with the client, or to join the group of workmates who take every opportunity to booze up when the company is paying. The issue with drinking at work functions is that in many situations, people do not really want to be drinking; they are drinking because it is expected of them. For those of us who are expected to attend work functions regularly, this tends to also mean that we are expected to drink regularly. What is crucial to remember is that this is not even social drinking, it is work drinking.

If such scenarios sound familiar, ideally you need to work towards feeling comfortable saying no to alcoholic drinks at work, or get very smart at managing these situations. For example, once you have said yes to the first offer of a drink, others tend to leave you alone, and there is no rule that you have to finish your drink once you have it. Simply take a few sips and then swap to water or other clear drinks so it looks like you are drinking. Human beings like to feel that they are the same as everyone else, so as long as you look as though you are drinking, you will find that others will leave you alone. If you are particularly strong and start to regularly say no when offered drinks, you will find others will lose interest and stop asking you altogether.

When it comes to making the best choice of alcoholic drinks there is no clear winner. Beer contains a high number of calories for the amount of alcohol you consume, and wine is sweet so it is easier to drink lots of it. Spirits are more concentrated and you can add low-calorie mixers to reduce the calorie content but these can be more difficult to get, especially when you are out at work functions. Overall, if you only drink occasionally, you do not need to be particularly fussy about what you are drinking. On the other hand, if you drink more regularly, a plain spirit with a low-calorie mixer is going to be a better choice, and leave you with less chance of a hangover.

Remember, work is work. It is not your life or your down time, and making the decision to keep your social life and work life separate is also a good way to keep an eye on your alcohol intake. The easiest way to take control of your intake is to have a drinking rule during the week, with no exceptions. You will then find that your weight and food intake during the week also start to take care of themselves fairly easily.

Snacking

For some, snacking is an important and regular part of their food day, while others enjoy 3 square meals a day. When it comes to the science, there is evidence to show that consuming small, regular meals and snacks every 3–4 hours can be beneficial to metabolic rate, and there is also evidence to show that individuals tend to regulate their appetite and caloric intake better when they consume 3 meals a day.

Experiencing hunger between meals is a good sign metabolically – it is an indicator that your body has burnt off the energy from the meal beforehand and needs more calories to continue burning efficiently. If you have eaten well-balanced meals with the right mix of carbohydrates and proteins, you should feel hunger 3–4 hours after that meal, usually in the late morning and late afternoon. This natural hunger mechanism can easily be deregulated when we eat our meals late, when we repress our hunger with coffee or when we are in the habit of skipping meals during the first half of the day and then eat continually throughout the afternoon. For this reason, a crucial aspect of taking control of your snacking habit is to take control of your mealtimes. Once you are eating your breakfast early in the day and lunch before 1pm, you will find you are only likely to need a small snack midmorning and a filling, protein-rich snack between 3 and 4pm to take you through until dinnertime.

Next, you need to know how to choose the right snacks so that when you do feel genuinely hungry, your snack choices will keep you full for the next few hours. A simple thing to consider when you select a snack is that it needs to be thought of as a 'mini meal', and as such it needs to keep you full for at least 2 hours. So, next time you feel peckish and take a look at a couple of biscuits or a packet of chips, ask the question: 'Will this keep me full for a decent amount of time?' If the answer is no, there are better choices to be made.

Generally speaking, a nutritious and filling snack food option will contain a mix of slowly digested, or low-glycaemic index carbohydrates for energy, as well as protein for fullness. Aiming for this combination of food groups not only ticks a number of boxes nutritionally, but it also automatically eliminates a number of processed snack food options such as rice crackers and snacks, muffins, biscuits, cakes, pastries and chips, which tend to be high in rapidly digested carbohydrates while offering little nutritionally.

If you like to check the nutrition labels of the foods you are purchasing, ideally a snack will contain <1000kJ per serve and between 10 and 20g of total carbohydrates; at least 5–10g of protein and <3g saturated fat per 100g. Remember that although nuts and the products that contain them appear very high in fat, much of the fat is unsaturated. Unsaturated fat, when consumed in small quantities, is known to have a number of health benefits and hence nuts and nut-based snacks are still good choices, as long as they are consumed in controlled portions. Lighter snacks of between 100 and 150 calories are the best choices in the morning when it may only be an hour or two before lunch, and more substantial 150–200 calorie snacks with 10–20g of protein will help keep you full until dinnertime.

Great snack food options for busy people include reduced-fat cheese and wholegrain crackers, thick yoghurts with fruit, skim milk-based drinks, nut- and protein-based snack bars and protein drinks. Packaged options including nut-based snack bars are easily kept in cars, briefcases and handbags to ensure that you are never caught out without something decent to munch on, so you can avoid the high-fat snack food options traditionally found at coffee shops, airports and in hotels.

❉ *While fruit is a nutritious snack choice, it does not contain any protein, so always team your fruit snack with some cheese, nuts or natural yoghurt.*

As part of your commitment to the Monday to Friday Diet, get into the habit of always having a protein-rich snack choice on hand to deal with hunger should it arise. Some standard snack choices are listed here, as are some more ideas in each of the daily plans.

Top snack choices

Nut-based snack bar

4 grain crackers with cheese

Small skim latte

100g thick yoghurt and berries

2 corn crackers with cottage cheese

½ cup edamame beans

2 cups popcorn

A protein shake or bar

2 rye crackers with goat's cheese and tomato

Small serve of hummus with vegetables

Focus on the vegetables

The funny thing about health, nutrition and weight loss is that if people simply prioritised eating more vegetables and salad on a daily basis, far fewer of us would have weight issues. The reason for this is that the majority of vegetables, with the exception of potato, sweet potato and corn (which are carbohydrate-based) have virtually no calories, which in turn means that you can basically eat as much of them as you like.

Adults require at least 2–3 cups of vegetables or salad every single day to get all of the fibre, bulk and numerous nutrients that brightly coloured vegetables offer. And yet, busy people are often getting less than half this amount on any given day. In fact, if you do not include a salad or soup at lunchtime, chances are you are getting nowhere near the amount of vegetables that you ideally need on a daily basis.

So in your quest to take control of your working week, a crucial component is focusing on eating more vegetables and salad during your day. This means making sure that your lunch is based around vegetables, whether this is via soup, salad or leftover veggies, and snacking on at least one vegetable each day. Vegetables make the perfect snack. They are generally not sweet, so you are not tempted to eat more and more of them. They are bulky, so they fill you up. They have virtually no calories but are so rich in nutrients that they are one of the few types of food that are actually linked to a reduced risk of developing some types of cancer in the long term.

So next time you go to grab a piece of fruit or muesli bar as you try to be 'healthy', grab a vegetable instead. Your health, your weight and your tummy will benefit in the long term.

VEGETABLE/SALAD (PER CUP, RAW)	TOTAL CARBS (G)	TOTAL CAL
Broccoli	<1	20
Pumpkin	10	70
Carrot	7	45
Tomato	4	30
Red capsicum	4	30
Cucumber	3	16
Peas	10	100
Green beans	3	30
Beetroot	10	60
Celery	1	15

Lunches

❖ *Do not underestimate the importance of lunch in weight control.*

People underestimate the power of lunch in their quest for long-term weight control. A lunch eaten too late is likely to have you crave sugar and overeat throughout the evening; while a lunch with the wrong balance of carbs, proteins and vegetables will most likely leave you unsatisfied for the remainder of the afternoon. For busy office workers, it is common for lunch to be delayed until 2 or 3 in the afternoon, while for mums there is often just not enough time to fit in a decent lunch before the school pick-up. Whatever the reason for your lack of lunch balance, if you are serious about your body and your weight, it is time to take your lunch more seriously.

Timing is so important when it comes to our food intake – ideally, we need 3–4 hours between meals to let our digestive hormones return to normal and allow the body's natural hunger and fullness signals to work optimally. What tends to happen in modern life is that regular snacking and coffee drinking disrupts these natural mechanisms and we do not experience the distinct hunger signals that we once did. Since we are often not hungry at lunchtime, we skip it or leave it until much later in the afternoon, when we snack and pick until dinnertime.

To take control of this daily pattern and the negative weight-gain cycle that results, lunchtime needs to be made a priority and it also needs to be nutritionally balanced. Ideally, you need to eat lunch by 1pm and make sure that it ticks the 3 nutritional boxes: carbohydrates for energy, protein for fullness, and salad and vegetables to help keep you full throughout the afternoon. A couple of pieces of sushi or a plain sandwich will not cut it; your lunch should be almost as filling as dinner and keep you full and satisfied until at least 4pm.

The lunch rules

1. Eat your lunch by 1pm each day.

2. Always eat lunch away from the kitchen or desk, and take 20 minutes to eat it.

3. Make sure your lunch contains the 3 core components: carbohydrates, proteins, and salad or vegetables.

4. Finish your lunch with herbal or black tea to cleanse the palate.

5. Try to walk around for at least 20 minutes after you eat to aid digestion.

The smart way to eat out

❁ *Eating out is a normal part of the week for many people and hence we have to know how to manage our food choices when we are eating out.*

Increasingly busy lifestyles, long working hours and numerous daily commitments mean that eating out has become a routine part of modern life. Unfortunately for those who enjoy a restaurant meal, eating out is likely to mean extra kilojoules thanks to the mix of larger portion sizes, the heavy use of oil, butter and rich sauces as well as numerous courses. Here are my top tips for eating out without gaining weight.

Choose your cuisines carefully

Indian, Chinese and Thai food in particular tend to be extremely high in fat due to their overuse of high-fat sauces such as coconut milk and batters, as well as the large volumes of oil used for frying a range of menu options. When high-fat curries and fried foods are eaten in conjunction with large amounts of white rice, noodles and breads, it is easy to see how a kilojoule overload can result. Ideally, such high-fat cuisines need to be consumed sparingly, just once or twice a month.

Look for the light options

Japanese, Greek and even Modern Australian cuisines tend to have a much wider range of menu items that will allow you to make healthier choices. Any sort of raw fish, grilled meat or seafood will be a great choice, especially when teamed with a large portion of vegetables or salad.

Size is everything

The truth is, if we simply ate smaller portions of everything, far fewer of us would have a weight problem. We don't really need both an entree as well as a main course, and for most of us an entree-sized portion of heavier foods such as pasta or risotto will be more than sufficient. If the serving of pasta, rice or meat is larger than you need, before you start your meal, visualise how much of the portion you plan to eat and take the excess off your plate and share it with your fellow diners.

When it comes to desserts, no one is saying that you have to avoid them completely. But remember that most of the pleasure of a dessert is gained in the first few mouthfuls, so if you really spot something you love on the menu, share it with as many people as possible.

Vegetables, vegetables, vegetables

One the biggest issues with meals consumed away from the home is that they rarely contain the amount of vegetables or salad that we need for good health and to help us feel full and satisfied. Even though vegetables can be expensive when ordered as sides, it is worth ordering extras to help bulk up your meal so you are not tempted by extra chips or bread.

Dealing with longer and longer workdays

❧ *Forget an 8-hour work day; nowadays if you factor in commuting you are lucky if you are home before you have given 12 to 14 hours to your work day.*

The fact that so many people struggle with their food choices and maintaining a regular exercise commitment comes as no surprise when you consider how much time people spend at work each day. Long gone are the days when we waltzed into the office at 9am and were well and truly gone by 5pm. Now we are lucky if we start the working day as late as 9am, and we tend to still be in the office until 6pm at the earliest. From a weight control perspective, long working days pose numerous issues.

First of all, for many of us long working hours equate to long periods of time sitting down. Metabolically, this is one of the worst things you can do as the cells become less and less efficient at burning calories the longer you spend sitting down. Then there is the boredom associated with spending many hours in the same environment, so we are more likely to look towards food for comfort and distraction. Long working hours can also mean that you become a victim of the environment in regards to food availability and the meals and snacks you have access to throughout the day. Unfortunately, few offices have access to the calorie controlled, low-fat, nutrient-dense foods that most of us need to keep our weight on track.

The rather harsh reality is that few of us are able to change the fact that we need to spend longer hours than we once did to get ahead at work. This means that if we also want to stay in control of our weight, we need to establish strong habits to ensure we remain in control of our working environment rather than it taking control of us.

Monitor your weight

One of the simplest things you can do when it comes to weight control is to keep an eye on your weight, week in, week out. Getting into the habit of stepping onto the scales regularly will help to inform you when things are starting to creep up and, in turn, when you may need to cut back. This is of particular importance when you are starting a new job or shiftwork, because a change in routine can see your weight increase very quickly.

Know your food basics

Although you are spending more time at work, this does not necessarily mean you need any more calories. In fact, it may actually mean the opposite: that you need fewer calories simply because you are sitting down more. The simple food rules of always eating a protein-rich breakfast early, aiming for lunch by 1pm and eating as early a dinner as possible will serve you well, no matter how many extra hours you find yourself at your desk.

Do not keep food on your desk

Sure, it is a good idea to keep nutritious snacks on hand, but if it means that you are eating more and more simply because the snacks are readily available, it may not be the best idea. Keep your snacks in a place where you at least have to get up to retrieve them, or you risk eating more simply because the food is in front of you.

Stick to your eating and non-eating times

A food rule that will serve you well during your entire working career is to only eat when you are hungry, or at least if it is a defined meal or snack time. The structure will help you to plan your workday and ensure that you do not fall into mindless eating when food crosses your path.

Ask for what you want

It does not matter if you are at a conference, on a course or staying in a hotel, feel confident in seeking out the food you need to have access to in order to keep on track with your diet. Salads, lean proteins and vegetables do not have to be that difficult to find but if we never ask for them and always eat what is provided, we continue to be victims of our food environment rather than in control of it.

Keep away from feeders

Feeders are interesting people. While they may seem kind and caring, they can also be a major source of calories and weight gain if we are not careful. Identify potential feeders in your office and learn to be comfortable in saying no to their kind high-calorie food offerings, which they, funnily enough, often do not eat themselves.

Accept and move forward

Some aspects of our working week simply cannot be altered. We have to be at work during certain hours, or we have various commitments at home and may only be able to exercise on certain days of the week. Now, we can choose to become frustrated by these limitations or accept things as they are and work within our own limitations to do the best we can with the hours and options that we have.

Make an effort to move

You may not have sufficient time to exercise but you can still make an effort to move as much as you can during the working day. Get off the bus or train one stop earlier, walk to work if you can, walk up and down stairs and escalators, and move around the office. Every little bit helps during the weekday.

Get out at least once a day

No matter how many hours you have to work each day, if you do not prioritise movement and make a concerted effort to get out of the office each and every day, you will be facing an uphill battle when it comes to weight loss.

Consider change

Long working hours may be required in your job for short periods of time, or there may be other pay-offs that see you choose to stay in your current position, but long term, if your work is really impacting negatively on your health and wellbeing, it may be time to consider a change.

The art of compensation

❧ *Controlling your weight is not about knowing*
calories in versus calories out, it is about knowing
how to compensate when you have overdone things.

With an abundance of good-quality food and a personal life that
revolves largely around food and drink, it is to be expected that
at times we will overeat, especially if a definition of overeating is
simply eating when we are not hungry. While some people may be
able to adhere to a strict food regimen and diet for lengths of time,
inevitably at some point we all need to regulate our food intake
behaviour. This means knowing when to cut back, when to skip a
meal and what to do when we have overeaten so we can get back on
track physically and psychologically.

One of the most powerful ways in which we can do this is to know
how to compensate – in other words, to be able to adjust our food and
exercise behaviour in accordance with the amounts of food we have
been eating. This may be as simple as eating a light meal after a heavy
one, or going for an extra run when you have a big meal planned.
Or it could be doing a week-long detox after you have been celebrating a big event, or scheduling a series of personal training sessions for
those times when you know that will be the only way that you make
it to training.

Planning is one part of it, another is taking responsibility and understanding what you need to do in any given situation to regain control
over your own food intake behaviour. Another important aspect of

learning how to compensate is keeping a close eye on your weight. It is a known fact that one important habit of those people who lose weight and manage to keep it off is that they regularly weigh themselves to make sure their weight is not increasing. Self-monitoring your weight on a weekly, fortnightly or even monthly basis means that if you notice your weight is starting to creep up, you can quickly make the necessary adjustments to your lifestyle to keep it under control. Losing a kilo or two is relatively easy, but shifting 5 or 10 kilos that have crept on over several years can prove to be much more of a challenge. Hence the more closely you monitor your weight, without driving yourself crazy in the process, the better.

One way to start to compensate with your food intake is to make a concerted effort to eat a light meal after you have eaten a heavy one and, of course, to follow the rules set out in Reset Monday to help to compensate for big weekends. The next easiest and most simply compensatory action is to schedule in a little extra exercise around events where you know you are likely to overeat.

From a calorie perspective, here are some other ideas:

Exercise calorie counter

FOOD INTAKE	CALORIES IN	EXERCISE UNITS
Smorgasbord meal	600–800	2 hrs running
3-course meal with alcohol	1000–1200	4–6 hrs walking
Restaurant dessert	400–500	1 hr cycle class
200g block chocolate	1000	2 hrs cycling
175g packet of potato chips	900	3 hrs surfing
Large box of popcorn	540	1 hr swimming
Fast food meal	800–1000	1½ hrs stairs
Packet of lollies	680	3½ hrs yoga
Bottle of wine	510	45 mins aerobics
Pie at the footy	450	40 mins X-trainer
Piece of cake at work	250	20 mins sprinting

When you are not feeling 100%

❀ *I am just so tired all the time.*

We have pills to relieve a cold, a migraine headache and to help us sleep, but unfortunately there is nothing we can take that will eliminate fatigue. Many of us live with fatigue on a daily basis.

Why are we all so tired? There are many reasons. We can be tired from not getting enough sleep, from the demands of the kids, working too hard, dealing with weight issues or even from the guilt of not having enough energy to do all the things you need and want to do with the day.

This is not surprising. So many of us have frantic lives with long working days and even longer commutes, ever-increasing family and relationship commitments and bumper social lives that mean it is a constant juggling act to get through the day, let alone with a reasonable amount of rest and time to get our thoughts together to power on all over again. While the demands of modern life are unlikely to change anytime soon, there are a few key lifestyle changes you can commit to that will at least help maintain your energy levels on a daily basis so you cruise to the end of your day, rather than collapse into it.

Iron up

If you are a meat eater you need to eat red meat 3–4 times each week. Why? Simply because your body is programmed to absorb the iron it needs to transport oxygen around the body from animal sources of iron, namely red meat. If you do not give your body regular access to it, your stores will gradually be depleted and you will be tired. Vegetarians are different, as they are programmed to absorb their iron from non-meat sources. But meat eaters, you need that steak, lamb or pork 3–4 times every single week.

Get into the sun

While you may not be keen to bring on any more wrinkles, the truth is that many Australians are simply not getting enough sunlight to ensure they are making adequate vitamin D. This vitamin has numerous functions in the body, and is also known to help prevent a number of diseases including some types of cancer. When it comes to energy levels, low vitamin D also tends to result in lower mood states and muscle fatigue, so if you are not feeling 100% and cannot remember the last time you went out into the sun, it may be time to have your vitamin D level checked by your GP.

Fresh is always best

For busy women on the run, grabbing a one-off coffee, protein bar or pre-made sandwich in place of a home-prepared, nutritious snack is not an issue. But if your diet is based solely around processed foods and supplements, you will not be doing your energy levels or immune system any favours. Fresh foods include fruits, grains, vegetables and seeds, which offer numerous nutritional benefits over any processed foods. This means you need these foods every single day to keep your training body at its best. As a general rule of thumb, the brighter the fresh food the better it will be for you, and we need at least 2–3 cups of brightly coloured vegetables and a couple of pieces of fruit every single day. Easy yet convenient ways to get your vitamin hit each day include grabbing a fresh juice rather than a coffee, keeping quick-cook vegetable packs at work and at home for quick dinners, and snacking on fresh carrot sticks and other cut up vegetables on a daily basis.

Watch the stimulation

The ironic thing about consuming caffeine and other 'energy'-type drinks to help increase energy is that they are just as likely to leave you feeling even worse than before you consumed them. The reason for this is that although stimulants, whether they are in the form of caffeine or sugar, will give you an initial 'hit', they will be followed by a subsequent 'drop' once the stimulant has been metabolised. For this reason, using caffeine in small amounts regularly and avoiding all sugar-based drinks is a much better option than relying on them for an energy hit in times of trouble. Ideally, large volumes of water, some herbal tea and a couple of cups of tea or coffee each day are the best types of fluid for you to ingest to keep you optimally hydrated and your energy systems at their best.

Add in your energy superfoods

When energy demands are high, it makes sense to include as many nutrient- and energy-rich foods in your diet as you can. Often, when women try to keep their weight down they consciously drop carbohydrates from their diet, but it should be remembered that wholegrain carbs are a rich source of essential nutrients including the B group vitamins which are required for energy production. If you have been feeling tired, make sure that you are including at least one serve of wholegrain carbs in each of your meals and snacks.

Just as important is to ensure that you are getting plenty of powerful antioxidants from brightly coloured fresh fruits and vegetables on a daily basis. Add in a fresh vegetable juice and aim for serves of salad or vegetables at both lunch and dinner to fend off fatigue and give your body every chance of being at its best day in, day out.

Go to bed

Perhaps the most obvious and simplest way of improving your energy levels, preventing fatigue and feeling better in general is to simply get more sleep. While the average adult gets just 5–6 hours of sleep a night, we need as much as 7–9 hours to be at our best. So even if you can only get to bed early a few nights each week, make this commitment to yourself. Remove all electronic equipment from the bedroom, including mobile phones near the bed, and practise getting into bed by 10 or 11pm and reading before you sleep – just the way nature intended it.

Work and travel

❖ *It is so common for people to arrive at the airport and put on their holiday mindset where all food rules simply get thrown out the window and they drink and eat whatever they like.*

If we went on a holiday once each year this behaviour would pose no issue, but it is far more common for professionals to be travelling on a weekly basis as part of their work. Generally speaking, the food you find at airports and that is served on a plane is less than ideal nutritionally. It is either a high-calorie option from the food court or a high-carbohydrate meal on the plane, which is supposed to fill you up in small volumes with little thought for the fat or carbo-hydrate content or nutrition. Add to that the issue of flight delays, prolonged periods of waiting time of unknown duration and the fact that plane travel means you will be sitting down for relatively long periods of time and not burning many calories at all and it is easy to see how weight gain and work travel go hand in hand.

You have already lost half of your battle if you arrive at the airport for a work trip without knowing what you are going to eat and when. Finding yourself in a place where there are numerous poor food choices when you are hungry, you have time to kill and are bored, will inevitably mean that you eat things you never usually eat simply because they are readily available. It also means that you put yourself in a situation in which you have to make challenging food decisions in an environment where few good decisions are possible.

Or, once you are on board a flight, it means that you are only able to eat what food is available, and there are generally few good choices.

If you travel for work occasionally, it is not an issue – a burger here or there or a fatty snack will not be the end of your weight-loss efforts – but if this is a weekly occurrence it is time to take control and stop letting your work travel schedule prevent you from reaching your weight-loss goals.

Only eat at a mealtimes

It does not matter if you arrive at the airport at 5am, 3pm or 9pm, there are always people eating. Sure, it may be a mealtime in a time zone somewhere, but when you are going on short, interstate travel, chances are you are eating because you can, as opposed to actually being hungry. Keep control over your calories by sticking as closely to your regular mealtimes as you can. This may mean planning ahead and taking a sandwich with you, or keeping a meal replacement or protein bar in your briefcase or handbag to have on the plane or between flights; either way you always have a backup option ready to go should you need it. This may also mean saying no to a meal on a flight if it is not a meal time for you.

Eat as few carbs on the plane as possible

While the standard meal choices on a flight include noodles, rice, mashed potato and pasta, these have to be the worst foods to eat when you will be sitting for anywhere between 2 and 24 hours. Sure, you need to eat if it is a mealtime, particularly on long-haul flights, but be fussy with your choices and keep the fuel foods to a minimum. Pick out the vegetables and meat, enjoy the cheese and crackers and even a mini dessert, but steer clear of the heavy carbs – you will simply not be burning them while you are so sedentary.

Always carry a protein-rich snack with you

You can often track down fruit, crackers, muffins and muesli bars, but it is much harder to source protein-rich snack food options, particularly in-flight. For this reason, always carrying a protein bar, nut bar or other protein-rich snack food whenever you travel will mean that you have a backup on hand to manage your hunger without resorting to quick-fix, processed carbohydrate snack foods. While you may not need a snack, getting into a good habit of always carrying one with you means that you are never caught short, no matter how late a flight runs. And if you find yourself stuck without dinner, the best choice might be a protein bar and a coffee rather than a burger, pizza or other high-fat meal deal.

Know the best airport choices

When you are trying to take control of your weight, it is empowering to know what to eat and when, especially when eating out or if you are faced with a million different choices. This is particularly true of airports, where your food choices can be numerous or exceptionally minimal. Coffee is something you can track down at most airports and it is a food choice that does tend to keep you full. Wraps are another good choice, as are simple sandwiches; then you can usually find nut and protein bars where the books and magazines are sold. Again, the key foods to avoid when flying are the carbohydrate-heavy choices of fried food, pizza, pasta, muffins, cakes and pastries, which will basically sit in your stomach for however many hours you are flying.

No alcohol on the plane

Now this is not going to be a popular one, but the fact is that flying is already super stressful for the body, and adding alcohol simply places more stress on the various body systems. Alcohol exacerbates dehydration, is empty calories, and while a small amount may help you go to sleep in trips where you have multiple flights, chances are that you are going to feel far worse from having a drink than not.

The shiftwork challenge

❁ *When it comes to weight control, there is no harder challenge than shiftwork.*

If you have ever had to do shiftwork, you will be well aware of the challenges that working when you are supposed to be sleeping and sleeping when you are supposed to be working poses. Not only do you tend to spend much of your time tired, but constantly alternating your 24-hour clock as you rotate shifts tends to put your body in a continual state of confusion. On top of that, weight control becomes exceptionally hard. Often shiftworkers will eat to help stay awake, or manage the cravings that tend to rear their ugly head when we are tired. Less well recognised is the fact that our hormones are basically programmed so that we burn more calories during the first half of the day, while we store and build at night – hence the added issue of eating when we actually should be sleeping.

Putting aside these challenges associated with shiftwork, weight loss is not impossible. In fact, having a little more time through the week with whole days and big blocks of time off may make training and food preparation a little easier. The focus is simply a matter of getting organised and knowing what to eat when, so that you can reach your weight-loss goals, even as a shiftworker.

Stick to as normal an eating schedule as possible

Even though your daily schedule is running in reverse, your body does not know this, which means your metabolism and hormonal programming are still going to function optimally if you try to eat most of your calories during daylight hours and take in minimal carbohydrates and calories throughout the night. This will mean that you need to be fussy about the types of foods you eat while you are on night shift and simply shift your mealtimes slightly to fit in with your work hours.

For the most common shiftwork hours, in which you finish your shift in the early morning, at 6 or 7am, this translates to eating an early breakfast at work or once you arrive home and before you put yourself to bed. This should then be followed with a late lunch when you get up in the afternoon and then eating your evening meal before you leave for work, or at the beginning of your shift. Then, if you do feel the need to snack overnight, to either help keep you awake or because you are genuinely hungry, sticking to low-calorie, low-carbohydrate choices will help to control your calorie balance and give your body the break from eating that it needs overnight to resume its natural digestive balance.

Watch the saboteurs

One of the most commonly talked about issues with shiftwork is the influence of fellow workers bringing in or buying less than ideal food choices to either reward themselves for getting through a night shift or simply out of habit because that is what has always been done. Whether it is fast food – as that is the only thing readily available late at night – vending machine treats or home-baked goodies, it is easy to see how eating high-calorie, high-fat foods can easily become a habit when working night shifts.

While there is nothing wrong with an occasional sweet treat to help get you through a tough, long shift, the issue arises when these foods become a habitual part of shiftwork eating. Once a link between the work environment and a certain type of food is formed, it becomes harder and harder to break. Before you know it you are eating high-fat foods on every shift, which is why so many shiftworkers gain weight.

The only way to prevent this happening to you is to develop food rules that apply whether you are working on shift or not. This may mean that you do include a fast food meal or treat once a week when you are on shift, but for 80–90% of the time you keep your diet on track. To achieve this will mean getting organised and taking your food with you, only eating relatively close to mealtimes and having to say no to pushy coworkers. But it will also mean that you are far less likely to become a victim of shiftwork weight gain.

Do not use shiftwork as an excuse

There is no doubt that shift work is tough physically, mentally and emotionally, but it can also be very easy to start to use shiftwork as an excuse to not prepare your food, skip training sessions and eat badly. While shiftworkers may have several days of the week in which their schedules are turned completely backward, they also tend to have blocks of time off in which there is much time to get organised, prepare the food they need to eat well, and to exercise to make up for the times they skip sessions when they are working.

For all of us there will be times when work or family commitments take over and we cannot dedicate as much time as we ideally need to keep our lifestyle habits on track. Indeed, this may be the case when you have extended blocks of shiftwork. But then the opportunity to start over again will arrive when the next block of shiftwork comes around and you find that you have a little more time.

Be strict with your sleeping

Just as we need to be strict with our eating times and food choices on shiftwork, so too do we need to be strict with the times we sleep. As the body is already under significant stress from disrupted sleep patterns and working against the natural body clock, sleeping too little or too much can make it even more challenging to feel at your best during blocks of shiftwork. Scheduling blocks of sleep will make this easier to manage, as will timing your sleeping blocks so you do not end up oversleeping and wake feeling groggy and unrested. As a general rule of thumb, aim for sleeping at least a 6-hour block after a shift and no longer than 9 hours. If you still feel fatigued when you wake, you may benefit from a 1–2 hour catnap prior to starting work again.

Be strict with your exercise

For shiftworkers, exercise can actually be your best ally when it comes to making it through a block of shiftwork. Not only will exercise help to get the blood pumping after a daytime sleep block, but it will also compensate for nights when you have spent most of your time sitting in a comatose-like state.

Even if you can only manage a 20-minute walk the afternoon before you head off for shiftwork, that small amount of exercise during this period is better than nothing. Scheduling a personal trainer session or gym class will help enormously in maintaining your energy levels when you feel tired, and it will also give your shiftwork blocks some structure, rather than allowing you to fall into the pattern of working, sleeping, watching TV and going back to work.

There is no secret to maintaining motivation when it comes to exercise. It simply boils down to accepting that we all need to exercise regularly. If you are a shiftworker, it is likely that exercising even when you are tired will make you feel better, not worse.

Your days off are the perfect time to really ramp things up. When you have multiple days off in a row between rotating shifts, you also have the opportunity to make up for all the training sessions you have missed. As a starting point, commit to always training on your day off as it will help enormously in keeping your body in the best shape possible to be able to cope with the shiftwork long term.

Taking stock when things go wrong

Inevitably in life things do not always go to plan and, at times, no matter how organised or focused we are, unforeseen circumstances, both good and bad, disrupt the schedules and goals we have set for ourselves. Whether these disruptions are due to illness, family tragedy, financial restraints, job disruptions, marriages, new babies or disasters, it can become even more challenging to remain committed to health and fitness.

The worst thing you can do during such times is to beat yourself up over not eating as well as you may like to, or for skipping training sessions and gaining weight as a result – because the good thing about health, fitness and weight issues is that they are always there to work on when and if we are able to. Giving yourself a hard time will only make you feel worse, detract your energy from what is really important and, basically, achieve nothing.

When things are bad, the best thing you can do is focus on the small and seemingly insignificant things in your day that help you to feel a little better. Take time out to listen to some music, soak in a bath or sit quietly with a cup of tea – these simple pleasures will help to energise you when things are tough.

Individuals who are able to use slip-ups and stuff-ups to their advantage, to take stock, review and start over without holding onto resentment and frustration over the present moment (or even the past) will do well in the game of life. While our early programming and life experiences have a powerful influence over the way we initially react to less than ideal situations, the good news is that better coping systems can be learnt. Just as any habit requires focus, commitment and time to review and reprogram, so too does the ability to learn from situations that do not please us. Move on to acceptance and then build new action plans from there.

This is especially true when it comes to slip-ups while you are attempting to reprogram your diet, exercise and lifestyle habits. Shifting your mindset from, 'Stuff it, I have blown it now', to one of, 'What is the best thing I can do from here to move forward?' will help you gain perspective and appreciate that one slip does not mean all is lost, and the best thing you can do is to table active steps to move forward.

Busy Businessmen

❁ *For you to do well in the boardroom you need to*
look after your weight, your body and your health –
then your performance can be at its best.

Unlike women, men tend to be far less food focused. On the one hand this may be perceived as a good thing – the less you think about food, the less you eat and the better it is for weight control, right? Not necessarily. When men fail to eat an adequate number of calories and key nutrients during their working day, they then tend to overeat later in the day, which can mean they are prone to significant weight gain in the long term.

Now, while a robust businessman is the image we commonly hold of a powerful, successful man, from a health and lifestyle perspective there are many downsides to this picture. Whereas a couple of kilos may not hold you back too much, once you are carrying around an extra 10–20 kilos, your energy is likely to suffer. You are more likely to experience sleep apnoea, which will be preventing you from getting good quality sleep, as well as health risk factors, including heart disease and diabetes. Often men can forge on with various health-related issues for many years but it is safe to say that even though they may be getting through their day, they are unlikely to be feeling or performing at their best.

The stressful, high-pressure world of a high-level worker is one thing, but the effect this stress can have on the body is phenomenal. Back pain, joint pain, headaches, fatigue, heart palpitations and high blood pressure are just some of the symptoms busy business-men live with on a daily basis, like a ticking time bomb waiting to explode. Some men may live like this for many years, continually pushing their physical limits and hoping for the best. Some of them will make it through but others will not, with heart disease, depression, cancer or interpersonal issues such as marriage breakdowns and relationship issues rendering any work success meaningless in the grand scheme of things.

Even for the highest functioning executives, health and nutrition can go off track due to a number of factors. Relentless schedules and time demands, regular international and interstate travel, and a lack of understanding and appreciation for the ways in which a healthy lifestyle can actually help workplace performance long term are just some of the issues. In fact, if executives operating in a high-level career appreciated how much better they would work, look and feel if they simply made it a priority to eat well and factor exercise into their schedules, it would be a no-brainer for them.

Skipping breakfast

Men are notorious for skipping breakfast, simply as they are often itching to get to work and do not understand that feeling hungry throughout the morning is actually a good thing metabolically. The issue with skipping breakfast is that not only do you fail to give your metabolism the kick-start it needs each day, but skipping breakfast has also been shown to result in you eating most of your calories during the second half of the day and gaining weight as a result. It does not matter whether it is a breakfast shake, egg sandwich or a quick bowl of cereal, you need to eat breakfast every day, and the earlier the better.

The breakfast meeting

For many executives, the working hours of the day are so long that breakfast meetings can occur as often as 3–4 times each week, and that can mean eating a whole lot of pastry. Keep your key food rules at the forefront of your mind and make a concerted effort to avoid the high-fat 'treat' foods so commonly served at buffet-style events. Instead, look for the protein-rich options of eggs, smoked salmon and lean meats teamed with low-fat milk, cereal and fruit to keep you fuelled throughout your day without the extra fat and calories that are unlikely to be burnt if you sit at a desk for most of the day.

The work lunch

The work lunch is the meal in which your diet goals tend to fall off track. While prepared wraps, sandwiches and hot food chosen from restaurants may not look to be poor choices, rarely do they contain the nutritional profiles that are optimal for weight control. Rather than being high in carbohydrates and inadequate in both protein and salad vegetables, work lunches need to be light yet filling to help sustain your blood glucose level throughout the afternoon. Good choices include sushi with seaweed salad, bean and tuna or chicken salads, meat and salad wraps or grilled fish and vegetables.

Drinks

The more senior the position, the more common it is for drinks to play a central role at work. Whether it is entertaining clients, work trips or attending conferences, even though it is 'work' you can find yourself drinking alcohol 3–4 times each week, and that is not taking into account the weekend. It is up to the individual to develop strategies in which they learn to regulate their drinking behaviour. Some may find they are better to not drink at all during the week, or to only have one drink. Others may find that as long as they control their carbohydrate intake, a couple of work drinks at any function cause no issue from a weight-control perspective. As a general health rule of thumb, adults need two alcohol-free days in a row each week and, for most of us, our health, sleep and waistline will benefit from a few more days alcohol-free than this.

Travel

Travelling tends to be a common aspect of any high-level management position, and in order for us to stay on top of our calorie intake and weight, some energy needs to be directed into making good choices at hotels and airports, otherwise weight gain is inevitable. Always travelling with protein-rich snacks is a good starting point, as is avoiding heavy carbohydrate-based meals when flying or participating in catered functions and events. Most importantly, factoring in exercise no matter where you find yourself on any work trip is a crucial part of maintaining a healthy lifestyle at home, interstate or overseas.

Business meetings

The catering at business meetings always seems to be the same – wraps, sandwiches, noodle boxes and fruit and cheese platters – but it is rarely what executives need to perform at their best. Lighter, more nutrient-rich options such as sushi, salads, and lean meat and vegetable options will not only keep an executive's energy up but, long term, they are also a must for weight control in a sedentary lifestyle.

The biscuit tin

If you skip breakfast, grab a quick lunch and are working until 8 or 9pm, chances are that if the biscuit tin crosses your path, you will be tempted. The issue with this is that nutritionally, cakes, biscuits and confectionery offer very little other than fat and calories, most of which are likely to be stored in the body if you spend most of your days sitting. Be strong; keep the lolly jar or biscuit tin out of sight and organise for healthier snacks such as fruit, cheese, nuts and protein bars to be kept on hand for those times when you need to eat, but need to eat something nutritionally balanced.

Coffee, coffee, coffee

It is common for busy businesspeople to drink coffee, or even tea, all day. The issue with this is that the constant stream of milk and possibly sugar to the cells cannot only put significant pressure on the liver but can also disrupt hunger and fullness signals so you skip meals during the day and then experience extreme hunger in the afternoon and evening. There is nothing wrong with enjoying a cup or two of coffee each day but always choose small coffees, drink more tea to reduce your caffeine intake and try to avoid adding much milk and sugar to keep down your calories.

Sitting down all day

If there is one thing that is worse for us than eating poorly and not exercising enough, it is sitting down all day. In fact, sitting down is the worst thing we can do for our metabolism as our cells become less and less efficient the less movement they do on a daily basis. For this reason, making a concerted effort to move as much as you can on any workday is crucial to not only help control your weight but to also protect your metabolism long term.

Keep up the medical checks

For busy executives, it can be surprising how quickly they let their basic health and fitness go if they do not get regular medical check-ups and manage such issues as high blood pressure, high cholesterol, low iron and low vitamin D. Make it a priority to have your blood tests routinely completed each year so you can stay on top of any health issues.

Schedule and pay for training

If there is one thing that executives understand, it is the importance of maintaining structure and schedules with effective time management. As we all need to exercise regularly, one of the best ways to ensure that this too becomes a natural part of your life is to book it in, pay for it and know that you see your trainer a certain number of times each week to give your body the workouts it needs to stay at its best, intense workday after intense workday.

Working Women

❀ *Want something done, give it to a working mum.*

Whether you work part time, full time or from home, the life of a working mum is nothing short of a constant juggle. And, even if you are an excellent juggler, chances are that you have little to no time for yourself, which means that eating and exercise are the first things that suffer when life is particularly frantic. The good thing about working mums is that they have to be exceptionally organised just to survive, and luckily they can use these organisational skills to also get their food and exercise on track, no matter how many hours they work, both paid and unpaid.

There is no group for which food preparation and organisation is more important than working mums. If you do not start your working week with at least two meals ready to go, and prepare your lunch the night before, the chances that you will eat well and be in control of your weight are slim. If, however, you get into a good habit of preparing as much food as you can for the week ahead, whether it be on a weekend or during the week, you will not only feel more in control of your life in general but also in control of your weight.

One of the key characteristics of women who lead frantic lives but who also manage to stay in control is that they utilise help around them. Whether it is the babysitter, their partner or outside help around the home, they contract out whatever they can afford to so that they can either be working or a mum or taking some time out, rather than trying to do everything. Naturally, the capacity to do this varies widely between individuals, but even if it means that you negotiate for your partner to give you one night off cooking each week, you are at least working towards being able to pull some time for yourself within your busy life.

Another common characteristic of efficient working mums is their ability to develop core structures and rules within their household so that things run smoothly. Whether it be no television during the week, strict bedtimes, set meals each week or quick meals on working days, these rules keep kids, husbands and staff in line so that they can get done what needs to be done in their busiest times during the week. Structures, rules and timetables help most of us, but even more so when our days are run by the minute.

Know your quick meals

When things are on track you may hope to have your meals planned and prepared for the week, but sometimes things will simply not go to plan. For nights when this happens you need to know what healthy meals you can make in 10 minutes. Whether it is a BBQ chicken with vegetables, frozen fish with a quick salad, or an egg and vegetable scramble, always have a list of meals you can prepare with the basic ingredients on hand so you can resort to them when you need to.

Always have a backup plan

This mantra tends to serve us well in many aspects of life but especially for when things do not come together. The concept of always having a backup plan – whether it is for dinner plans, a social event, the weather or what to wear – means that you are far less likely to be stressed, disappointed or upset when things do not go to plan.

'What if?' is always a good question to ask yourself so that these contingency plans are ready to go no matter what, and you're put in a much stronger position at times when things have gone haywire but you need to remain cool, calm and collected.

Use people

Highly successful, efficient people are often the least likely to ask for help, even when they really need it. Asking for help does not mean that you are using people – you simply need help to make your life a little easier. Whether it is your family, friends, your children's friends' parents or workmates, get comfortable with asking for a favour if you need it. Whether it is to help you pick up the children so you can make it to the gym, or asking your mother to babysit so that you have time to get a massage, constantly remind yourself that there is nothing wrong with asking for help if you need it. With every intention of also being able to return the favour, practise being comfortable enough to ask for help when and if you find that you need it.

Multi-task everything

Time for the working woman is everything, which means that making sure not a second is wasted can go a long way in ensuring that everything that needs to be completed on a daily basis is. Ironing while catching up on the phone, cleaning while cooking, or doing chores while helping with homework is not only likely to be the norm but a necessity to get you through the week.

Be smart with time

Here is a question for you: where do you waste time? Whether it is watching television and the advertisements that come with it, commuting during peak hour, shopping when the supermarket is at its busiest or simply talking on the phone, try to identify these times in your day and brainstorm ways to make these time wasters work better for you.

Get the kids working

There is nothing wrong with getting the kids to help at home. If anything, it teaches them that they too are an important part of the workplace called home, which needs constant servicing in order to keep running. Make a list of chores the kids need to do each day and have them help to prepare meals, fold laundry, make their beds and other routine jobs they could easily be doing so you can focus on more important aspects of your life.

Have clear time rules

Rules mean that everybody knows what they should be doing to keep a household running smoothly, at least during some days of the week. Rules will also ensure that you can create time for yourself because the kids are in bed when they should be, or the television is not acting as a distraction so you can more easily coordinate an active household on a daily basis. While each family will have different rules, develop ones for your own family, make everyone well aware of them and notice how much more smoothly things will run.

Schedule down time

For working women, down time may seem to be an unfathomable concept, but even if it is just 30 minutes each evening before you go to sleep or an hour on the weekend, schedule some time when you can switch off, sit and be calm to refocus and decompress from the frantic world that is your reality. Create a sacred space and time to do this and make it as calm and relaxing as possible – you may fall asleep but at least you had the time to switch off completely.

Listen to your body

Our bodies are exceptionally good at telling us what they need: headaches, fatigue, poor sleep and weight gain all are symptoms that we are not looking after ourselves in the way that we need to be at our best. Pay close attention to any signs or symptoms your body may be giving you as they are indications that you need to look after yourself a little better. Have blood tests done at least once a year and see your doctor when things do not feel 100%. Often all we need to get back to our best are some vitamins, more vegetables in our diet and more sunlight, but it is always better to be safe than sorry.

Know when to give yourself a break

Highly organised, efficient, high-achieving people not only tend to do well in life but they also tend to be very good at giving themselves a hard time, especially when things are not done perfectly. There is nothing wrong with having high standards, in fact they are likely to have got you to where you are today, but knowing when to lay off a little and give yourself a break is an important part of being human. Life is hard enough without you giving yourself a hard time as well.

Seek out those who support you

It is a good idea to be smart with people in general and make sure that the core group you have around you, whether it be friends or family, are indeed those people who nourish your soul and help you to be the best you can be. Life is too intense to have people around you making things harder than they are already, so where you can, limit the time you spend with energy drainers and seek out the time and company of those who help you rather than bring you down emotionally or psychologically.

Prioritise sleep

The funny thing about sleep is that with just a little more of it, we are all likely to feel, look and function better. If you are regularly getting less than six hours' sleep a night, or often find yourself asleep on the couch in the early hours of the morning, it is time to take the elixir of sleep a little more seriously. Even if you can only manage it for 3 or 4 nights each week, make an effort to get into bed before midnight and remove any form of electronic stimulus in the bedroom. Not only will your relationship function better, so will your body.

For the mums

🌼 *The sooner a mother learns to look after herself, the sooner she will be a better mother.*

For those who have had children, few would argue against the notion that being a mother is perhaps the hardest job you can do. Not only are other people's wellbeing in your hands but on top of that you, will often also have a home and a partner to care for.

While there is no doubt that motherhood is a tough gig, not caring for yourself can only make it tougher. Skipping meals, eating the kids' leftovers and not prioritising your own exercise and sleep means that although your partner and kids may be doing well, the chances are that you are barely surviving. The weekdays are a frantic mess of rushing, driving, cooking, cleaning and delivering, while weekends are dedicated to the kids' and your partner's recreation time – a relentless and self-perpetuating cycle. No matter how exhausted you let yourself get, the chance that your husband or kids will even notice is slim. For this reason, your weekdays have to factor in some 'me' time to ensure that you do not get lost in your own life.

As is the case with any adult's schedule, whether they are a full-time or part-time worker, male or female, mother or not, getting on top of your week requires scheduling and organisation, and this also includes meeting your health and fitness needs. For many people, the common issue with planning comes when we overcommit and over-schedule ourselves. Instead of committing to just one or two gym sessions a week, we expect to get out of bed at 5am and go for a run or make it to the gym every single day, and then are disappointed with ourselves when we do not make it. A realistic and sustainable approach is to work on developing key routines that are factored in as a minimum 'must do' each week. Whether this is a set number of workouts, healthy lunches at home or time to cook and get organised, each will go a long way in reclaiming some time for you and getting your health and weight on track for the long term.

Schedule in your exercise time

Mums are notorious for 'allowing' things to get in the way of their opportunities to exercise – 'I had washing to do', 'Joey was sick', 'The day just got away from me'. There is no secret to ensuring that you exercise regularly, you simply have to prioritise and schedule it. For some mums this will mean exercising first thing in the morning, for others the evening is best or once their partner has arrived home, or it may mean committing to an exercise class or personal training appointment. Remember, while exercising every day would be ideal, you can still get good, sustainable results by committing to three good-quality training sessions each week. Start small and build from there with the goal of having at least 2 or 3 sessions factored into your schedule every single week – no excuses.

Commit to eating your meals

For many busy mums their day starts off on the wrong foot when they choose to feed the children before themselves, skip lunch in favour of coffee and find themselves binging at 3 or 4pm, once the school day finishes. As days with children, errands and activities are generally busy, and much time tends to be spent in the car, making sure that you begin each day with a protein-rich breakfast and allocating time for lunch is absolutely crucial to prevent over-eating in the afternoon.

Eat breakfast before you feed the kids

While a traditional approach from any mother is to feed the children before she feeds herself, especially at breakfast, it can be argued that mums will be in a much better position both physically and hormonally if they eat their breakfast as soon as they get up in the morning, rather than feeding the children first. Not only is eating breakfast as early as possible crucial for weight control, but actively showing children that mum and her needs are just as important as theirs is an important thing for kids to learn.

No kids' scraps

Picking at leftovers and snacking during food preparation tends to be a dietary issue for all of us, but even more so for mothers who have not eaten well and then find themselves nibbling all day on the kids' food. Half a sandwich here, a few biscuits there and before you know it, you have eaten an entire extra meal's worth of calories. Be mindful of where extra food may slip into your day and make a concerted effort to only eat at a meal or snack time rather than grazing on food when you may not even be all that hungry.

Only one dinner

Long working days mean that many families operate with two dinnertimes: an early dinner for younger children and then another dinner later in the evening once the children are in bed. The issue with this is that mums tend to be hungry way before their second dinnertime at 8 or even 9pm and eat a little at the earlier dinner and then again with their partner later in the evening. Be aware of this being an issue from both a calorie and digestion perspective, as it really is better to eat your main meal before 8pm.

Watch the coffee dates

Women love to meet over coffee, which is not a problem unless 'coffee' regularly becomes multiple coffees and cakes to match. It only takes one member of the coffee club who enjoys a sweet treat with her coffee to encourage all members to go off track with their diets. For this reason, be mindful of not only how often you have coffee with friends, but also what you are eating as part of that experience.

Daily time out with self

Taking time out, even just half an hour to do what you want to do can be one of the most difficult things for busy mothers to add into their schedule. Time for self is imperative, not only to maintain some sort of sanity in the chaotic world in which mothers find themselves but also to be able to do the things you need to do to look and feel at your best, whether it is to phone a friend, get a pedicure or simply sit down and read a magazine uninterrupted. While creating this time may require some negotiation with your partner, or investing in a babysitter, the health and wellbeing benefits you will gain will be well worth it.

Time out with your partner

When was the last time you managed to take some real time out with your partner, such as a whole evening or weekend to recon-nect, spend some quality uninterrupted time together and remind yourself of why you liked your partner in the first place? With such little time spent together and the pressure on modern families, is it any wonder that relationships break down? If you value your family life, and know that the most important relationship in your life needs more time, start to schedule a regular date night and weekend away. You will be surprised what a difference quality time together makes in any relationship.

Once you have regained control of your weekdays

❀ *I long for the days when life was simple: work finished at 5pm, weekends were for relaxing and I seemed to have so much more time.*

The sad thing about modern life is that many of us have forgotten how to live. Instead, we exist on a daily basis and the things that are most important to us, the aspects of our lives that give us the most meaning – nurturing our souls, relationships and passions – are left to slowly disappear, leaving us wondering where things went wrong.

While the pressures and demands of life are unlikely to change – if anything they are likely to become more intense – the secret to rising above the slog of life is to regain control over our days. Once we actively decide to manage our days, time and resources, no longer are we victims of our lives but we are living them. And, most importantly, we are living them with meaning.

Taking care of our bodies and our minds by eating good food, getting regular exercise and caring for ourselves forms the basis of this ability to feel well, look well and be able to perform well on a daily basis. *The Monday to Friday Diet* has been written to help you build your own platform on which to do this. My hope is that it will help you to thrive and flourish throughout all your working days to come.

Also by Susie Burrell

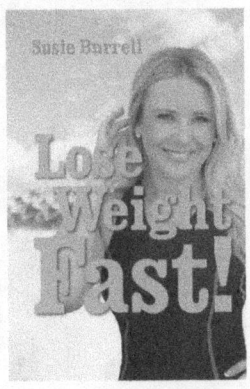

Do you need to shift some weight for an upcoming event? Are you sick of being on a calorie-controlled plan with no real outcome? Have you tried every diet, lost a couple of kilos and then reverted back to your old lifestyle habits? Would you like to know how to kickstart fat-burning when you need it most? *Lose Weight Fast!* is the weight-loss guide you need to help manage your weight-loss goals now. With tips and tricks, meal plans and recipes that show you how to lose one, ten or even twenty kilos as quickly and safely as possible, you will finally have the tools you need to get rid of the weight, the right way.

Now available as an ebook.

Loved the book?

Join thousands of other readers online at

AUSTRALIAN READERS:

randomhouse.com.au/talk

NEW ZEALAND READERS:

randomhouse.co.nz/talk

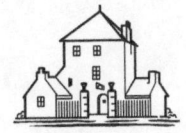